Newborn Essentials:

A Parent's Guide
to
Best-Evidence Baby Care

J. Wells Logan, MD

Name: J. Wells Logan, MD
Title: Newborn Essentials: A Parent's Guide to Best-Evidence Baby Care
Identifiers:
ISBN: 979-8-9909936-1-7 (paperback)
       979-8-9909936-2-4 (e-book)

Published by Newborn Essentials, LLC

St. Johns, FL

Newborn-Essentials.com

CONTENTS

PREFACE: A LIFE-CHANGING JOURNEY

For some, the prospect of caring for a newborn is the fulfillment of a lifelong dream. For others, the notion that a small, defenseless baby will soon rely on them for survival is simply overwhelming! Whatever your background or perspective, a baby changes everything! The birth of a newborn heralds the beginning of a lifelong journey; and while this journey has its challenges, it is also among life's most meaningful and rewarding experiences. So, if caring for a baby is in your future, then you embark on an incredibly important pilgrimage—and the book in your hands has the tools you need to make it successful!

This handbook of newborn essentials provides three important aids for your journey. First, you will learn the importance of providing a safe, nurturing home environment—one that supports healthy newborn development. Second, you will learn to manage the most common challenges of the newborn period, with confidence and ease. Third, and perhaps more importantly, you will learn the fundamentals of newborn health and well-being—concepts that are important throughout the first year. What distinguishes this book from so many others, however, is that each concept is supported by evidence from the medical literature. Here you will learn not only how to care for a newborn, but *why* each concept is important, and *when* to be concerned. And while these concepts are essential, the good news is that they can be easily learned and applied to a wide range of circumstances. In the time it takes to read this book, you will learn to provide safe, developmentally appropriate care for your newborn and in so doing, you will find yourself less anxious and better able to enjoy this memorable induction into parenthood.

Before we begin, however, consider three important disclaimers. First, this book is intended to supplement, not replace, the care of your pediatrician. No book, workshop or website can replace a good pediatrician. So, if at any point in your journey you become concerned about your baby's health or safety, please put the book down and call your pediatrician! Second, these concepts are unapologetically honest. Although most newborn conditions are benign or inconsequential, newborns do occasionally fall ill—just like the rest of us. As such, selected newborn conditions are included so that you are better able to recognize the *early* signs of illness, and how to distinguish these (and other *potentially avoidable* complications) from those that are benign or inconsequential. Third, this book arises from the Judeo-Christian view that every child is made in the image of God. Therefore, every child has intrinsic beauty and worth, regardless of his/her stage of development and physical or intellectual capacity. If you can accept these provisions, then we will have enough common ground for the discussion that follows.

By now you may be asking, "What, exactly, is the *newborn period*, and why is it so important?" The term *newborn* generally refers to the first three to four months of life, but the emphasis here is on the first six months—a critically important period in child development. In reality, the concepts included here are true of older infants as well, but the application of these concepts is so important in the first six months that they deserve special consideration. As a newborn physician (neonatologist), I admit some bias regarding the importance of newborn care, but I think you will soon agree that these principles are important. Moreover, understanding these concepts will prove a valuable resource throughout the first year.

We begin Part I with the fundamentals—providing a safe, nurturing home environment for mother-infant bonding and nutrition. We then explore the benefits and challenges of breastfeeding—on bonding, growth, and early brain development. Because brain growth peaks in the first six months of life, chapter 3 considers the important link between the quality of human interactions and early brain development. In chapter 4, we examine common pregnancy complications, and how these impact the transition from fetal to newborn life and briefly discuss the principles of early postnatal care. Chapter 5 examines the transitional period in more detail, how it relates to discharge readiness, and the hospital pre-discharge screening process. In chapter 6, we review conditions that are commonly encountered soon after delivery, especially those that can delay hospital discharge. Part I concludes with chapter 7—an examination of common but generally benign conditions experienced in the first six months. Throughout the book, the emphasis is on healthy, full-term newborns, as the vast majority of infants are born between 39- and 40 weeks gestation, with all the usual signs of health and well-being.

Part II explores the more challenging aspects of newborn care. For example, as many as 12 percent of pregnancies result in premature labor and delivery; so chapter 8 is devoted to the care of infants born preterm.[1] Sudden unexpected infant death is rare, by comparison to prematurity, but a potentially avoidable threat to the newborn, so chapter 9 is given to recognizing and minimizing known risk factors.[2] While birth defects and disabilities are largely unavoidable, the prevalence of disabilities appears to be increasing. Therefore, chapter 10 includes an evidence-based discussion of infants born with birth defects or disabilities.[3, 4] We conclude Part II with a summary of important concepts and some practical ways you can prepare for the journey. Part III is for those who want a deeper dive into newborn medicine. Appendix A provides a brief summary of conditions that warrant a formal evaluation by a pediatrician and Appendix B, a brief summary of the most common birth defects.

Fortunately, the vast majority of conditions encountered in the newborn period are benign or uncomplicated - requiring only supportive care or observation. Nonetheless, the signs of illness are often subtle in the newborn period, so the ability to recognize the signs of illness is fundamental to newborn care. Thus, you will learn to distinguish between a wide array of harmless conditions and those that require the attention of your pediatrician. In this way, you will gain the confidence and assurance needed to provide safe, developmentally appropriate care for your precious baby.

Inspired by hundreds of conversations with family and friends and over 25 years of clinical practice, this volume provides the guidance you need to navigate the challenges of the newborn period, safely and effectively. Your grasp of these concepts will be rewarded with the peace of mind that comes from understanding what is important, *and what is not*, in the care of your newborn. I suggest reading one chapter at a time, pausing long enough to reflect on key concepts. The book is intentionally brief to emphasize important concepts, which are easily lost in the "noise" of the unimportant.

Finally, please visit our website at newborn-essentials.com for more information about the book, its author, and fresh content related to newborn care. If you like what you find, please sign up for periodic email alerts, and share the link with family and friends who share your passion for newborn care. Thank you for your interest and enjoy your journey through the newborn period!

J. Wells Logan, MD
St. John's, Florida
Dec 29, 2024

PART I THE FUNDAMENTALS

CHAPTER 1. FUNDAMENTAL NEEDS OF THE NEWBORN

The home environment plays an essential role in a child's overall development. Research has shown, for example, that healthy mother-baby interactions and age-appropriate stimulation play an important role in the formation of early brain connections.[5, 6] Consider, first, the importance of the home environment in terms of its impact on short-term health and well-being. A nurturing home environment is one that supports mother-infant bonding, allows for an uninterrupted feeding schedule, and includes the kind of stimulation that promotes early brain development.[7] Temperature regulation, a safe nurturing home environment, and healthy sleep habits all play an important role. Likewise, adequate nutritional intake and avoiding potentially dangerous exposures are fundamental to healthy newborn growth and development. Each of these concepts are discussed in brief as *fundamental* needs of the newborn.

Temperature Regulation

In the first days and weeks after birth, newborns are vulnerable to both heat and cold stress. The temperature control centers in the developing brain are relatively immature, and still adapting to postnatal life.[8, 9] Therefore, low (< 97.7°F or 36.5°C) core body temperatures suggest the baby is either cold stressed or ill (more on this later).[10-12] And what is true of full-term infants is especially true of infants born small for gestational age or premature.[13] The good news, however, is that cold stress can be avoided by simply keeping your newborn clothed and bundled in a thermally neutral environment. The evidence regarding elevated core body temperatures (*hyper*thermia) is mixed, so the American Academy of Pediatrics has refrained from making specific recommendations. However, there is some evidence that elevated environmental temperatures (e.g., over-bundling) can be harmful as well.[11, 14, 15] This is addressed in greater detail in chapter 9, but for now, let us establish that extreme temperatures, i.e., either cold or warm environments, should be avoided in the newborn period.

> Newborns need a warm, safe, nurturing environment for sleep, bonding, and early brain development.

Healthy newborns burn calories (energy) to maintain a normal core body temperature. Infants burn more calories in cool environments, leaving fewer calories (energy) for growth and weight gain. For example, a newborn who is kept in a room at 67°F will generally burn more calories (energy) to maintain a normal core body temperature than a newborn who is kept in a room maintained at 72°F. This is one of my pet peeves as a newborn physician. Too often, when rounding in the newborn nursery, I find that mother-baby pairs are bonding and breastfeeding in frigidly cold

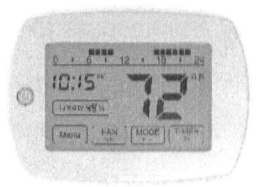

ID 37145874 © Lucadp | Dreamstime.com

hospital rooms. Given the risks of either extreme (temperatures ≤68°F or ≥75°F), I recommend setting the thermostat to a temperature that is somewhere in the middle (i.e., between 71°F and 73°F)—a thermally neutral environment. Preterm infants are especially prone to cold stress, and I have had the unfortunate experience of hospitalizing a set of preterm twins who became cold (hypothermic) during a routine pediatric office visit! Unfortunately, I had to take some ownership for this hospital admission, as the onset of hypothermia was due, almost assuredly, to being in a cool exam room (on a hot summer day). Overall, full-term newborns are less vulnerable to cold stress, as they usually have sufficient body mass (and brown fat) to regulate core body temperature in different environments.

Maintaining a normal core body temperature requires energy (calories) that can otherwise be used for growth. Therefore, using one to two thin blankets is recommended, and cotton is preferred, as cotton is more porous than synthetic fabrics. While the evidence is limited, most experts agree that over-bundling should also be avoided, to minimize the risk of accidental suffocation and overheating. The head/scalp is the largest surface area on a newborn's body and a significant source of radiant heat loss. After the first few days, the customary knitted cap is no longer needed and may lead to overheating. Likewise, in warmer environments, a single lightweight blanket is sufficient. If, on the other hand, you keep your home cooler than average (i.e., less than 70°F or 21°C), consider using at least two lightweight cotton blankets. Avoid ambient temperatures less than 68°F (20°C), as cool environments increase the risk of cold stress and poor weight gain. Most newborns tolerate lukewarm baths, but prolonged exposure to cool ambient temperatures should be avoided. Mottling of the skin is frequently observed in infants who are either cold or sick—but we will come back to this later.

Traveling with a newborn can be challenging in the summer and winter months, as newborns require more protection from the elements. It is wise, then, to prewarm (or precool) your automobile before travel excursions, beginning with your first trip home from the hospital. Minimize exposures to the elements and make contingency plans for unanticipated power outages that may affect home heating and cooling systems. If you live in a cool climate or an area where power outages are common, consider purchasing a home generator. Importantly, NEVER leave your newborn (or any child) in an unattended automobile! Each year, children die from heat exposure in unattended automobiles. On average, the ambient temperature in a closed automobile increases by 3.2°F every five minutes on a sunny day—even in the fall and winter months.[16] Newborns (and older infants) are also vulnerable to heat exposure, such as beach or poolside outings. Heatstroke is characterized by fever, lethargy, decreased urine output, excessive thirst, dry mucous membranes, and low neuromuscular tone (a floppy newborn). If your newborn has any one or more of these signs in the context of heat exposure, seek medical attention without delay.

A Safe, Nurturing Home Environment

A safe, nurturing home environment is essential for optimal newborn care, regardless of gestational age or birth weight. Research has shown that noise levels in the neonatal intensive care unit (NICU) contribute to abnormal development, and that the impact persists well beyond hospital discharge.[17] Likewise, a chaotic home environment can interfere with bonding, breast or bottle feeding, sleep, and healthy brain development.[18] While this may come across as common-sense advice, and indeed it is, the application of this principle is more challenging for some than for others. Maintaining a quiet, nurturing home environment is especially difficult for those who thrive on large crowds and social gatherings. Fortunately, just as newborns provide signals (cues) when hungry, cold, or wet, they also provide cues when overstimulated. Irritability (fussiness, excessive crying) is the most common sign of overstimulation. However, disorganized neuromuscular movements, yawning, and poor feeding habits are other signs of overstimulation. Loud music or television noise, for example, can interfere with one's ability to recognize these important cues, and this may have short- and long-term effects on newborn development. In a study designed to examine the impact of mother-infant interactions, mutual

> Research suggests that the home environment and mother-infant interactions can influence long-term health outcomes.

4

responsiveness in mother-infant pairs was associated with better language development and motor development in premature infants.[19, 20]

Human touch is fundamental to newborn development. Note, however, that researchers believe that optimal brain development depends on the *right kinds* of stimulation. Gentle rocking movements, light caresses, and soft embraces are practical ways to stimulate healthy brain development. Research suggests, for example, that positive, supportive experiences such as breastfeeding and skin-to-skin care are associated with stronger brain responses in newborns, while painful experiences, such as pinpricks or procedures, are associated with reduced brain responses.[21] In a study published in 2016, prolonged skin-to-skin contact was associated with earlier attainment of exclusive breastfeeding.[22] Similarly, a small study of Finnish newborns demonstrated that soft brush strokes applied to the skin during functional magnetic resonance imaging (MRI) scans activated brain regions linked with sensory and social processing.[23] Thus, positive, nurturing experiences, especially those related to human touch, appear to play an important role in early brain development.

Sleep is fundamental to newborn development. Establishing a consistent cycle of uninterrupted sleep is an important part of your parenting journey. Sleep/wake cycles are typically characterized by a period of sleep, followed by a period of arousal with hunger cues, and then again by a period of quiet contentment and alertness. Each mother/baby pair is slightly different, of course, but interruptions to this sleep/wake cycle can interfere with bonding, feeding patterns and growth, and may lead to *neurologic dysregulation*, a term used by physical and occupational therapists to describe an unhealthy neurologic state.[18] This suggests the importance of establishing healthy boundaries with family and friends, especially in the first few weeks of life, when bonding, sleep/wake cycles, and feeding routines are being established. Further, it is essential that your newborn develops these routines in a safe, nurturing, and developmentally appropriate environment. Family and friends play a vital role in a child's development and are an indispensable part of your support team. However, visits should be scheduled to minimize interruptions to this important routine. Anything that interferes with the mother or baby's routine is a potential threat to your newborn's health and well-being.

Safe sleep is essential to newborn well-being. The American Academy of Pediatrics has issued policy statements regarding safe sleep for newborns, as several *seemingly* harmless sleep habits are associated with an increased risk of sudden unexpected infant death (SUID).[11] The "Back to Sleep" program recommends that infants be placed on their backs (supine) for sleep, even for brief naps and between daytime feedings. This has become the *standard of care* in the US and is credited with significant improvements in infant survival.[11] In addition, the practice of swaddling should be discontinued at around six to eight weeks of age, or as soon as the newborn is capable of rolling from back to front (supine to prone). Swaddling after two months of age is believed to increase the risk of accidental suffocation, as is soft bedding and soft crib decorations (stuffed animals). Implementing safe sleep practices is one of the most important things you can do to provide a safe home environment for your newborn (more on this in chapter 9).

In summary, newborn development is related to a broad range of environmental and human factors, including environmental temperature, sleep/wake cycle, ambient noise, parental stimulation, human touch, human voice, and safe sleep practices. Positive, soothing words and social interactions, including eye contact, social smiles, and human touch, are important ways you can stimulate early brain development. Common sense is important here, as one need not walk around the house tiptoeing and whispering. Indeed, this could well be the *wrong* kind of stimulation. On the other hand, a chaotic home environment can produce sensory and environmental overload that interferes with feeding, bonding, sleep, and early newborn brain development. Importantly, responding to your newborn's basic needs by maintaining a safe, warm, nurturing home environment and recognizing hunger cues and signs of stress (crying/irritability), including soiled/wet diapers, are simple yet profound ways you can provide a healthy environment during this critical phase of development.

Nutrition, growth, and weight gain. Growth and nutrition are discussed extensively in the following chapter but are included here as they are among the most fundamental needs of a newborn. In the first weeks after birth, a full-term newborn is expected to gain between 20 and 30 grams per day, or five to seven ounces per week (30 grams ≈ one ounce or 1/16 of one pound). Most infants double their weight within five to six months and triple their weight by the end of the first year. Infants who fail to gain at least 15 grams (1/2 ounce) per day should be evaluated by a pediatrician or pediatric provider. Likewise, linear growth is an important marker of organ (e.g., heart, lung, brain) growth and development.[24-26] Infants usually grow 1.5 to 2 cm (3/4 to 1 inch) in length (stature) each month in the first six months of life and a newborn's head circumference increases by approximately one centimeter each month in the first six months. Fortunately, many of the challenges related to growth and nutrition have simple solutions and your pediatrician manages these challenges routinely—an important reason to establish a partnership with your pediatrician.

At the first post-discharge follow-up visit, your newborn's weight will be compared with the birth weight documented in the hospital discharge summary. Most newborns lose between 5 and 7 percent of their body weight in the first three to five days, only to regain this weight within 10 days of birth. If weight loss is excessive (> 10%), your pediatrician will explore potential causes and develop a plan to reverse the trend. Delayed breastmilk production is the most common cause of excessive weight loss but is typically transient and short-lived. Consultation with an experienced clinical lactation consultant or mother-baby nurse can provide the guidance and support needed, but follow-up (before and after discharge) is essential. Depending on the nature of the problem, supplementation with cow's milk formula may be needed, if only for a few days, while the mother's milk supply increases. Ongoing, persistent, or severe failure to thrive is uncommon but warrants consideration of cow's milk intolerance as a diagnosis (more on this later).

Avoiding Potentially Dangerous Exposures

As we close this chapter on the fundamental needs of a newborn, it seems appropriate to note that newborns are vulnerable to infection in the first few months after birth. Infections acquired during pregnancy (especially amniotic fluid infections) can lead to preterm labor and delivery, so newborns occasionally deliver prematurely with signs of infection. Even more rare is the infection acquired while passing through the birth canal. Infants who are deemed at risk, for one reason or another, should undergo diagnostic screening for infection after delivery. If risk factors are identified by the pediatrician or baby nurse, laboratory testing is appropriate, and a period of observation and/or treatment with antibiotics may be needed. The newborn immune system is relatively immature, and like other organ systems in the first days and weeks, is undergoing adaptation to postnatal life. Because the first set of childhood vaccines is not offered until the two-month well-baby visit, newborns are vulnerable to the most common community-acquired infections. Fortunately, the breastfed newborn gains passive immunity from maternal vaccination (before and during pregnancy) and from prior exposures to infection. Breastfeeding confers some protection against infections that might otherwise pose a greater risk to the newborn.

Handwashing and avoiding ill contacts can minimize the risk of infection.[27] Newborn infections typically present with one or more of the following signs: poor appetite (inadequate intake), decreased activity (lethargy), irritability (fussiness), or an abnormal temperature (≤97.7°F or ≥ 99.5°F). Fast breathing (tachypnea) and/or a rapid heart rate (tachycardia) are less subtle but more concerning signs of

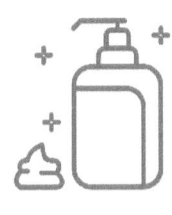

by haritselarif via Pixabay

infection and warrant an immediate evaluation by a pediatrician. However, any one of these signs of illness should prompt an evaluation. The presence of other clinical signs, such as vomiting, diarrhea, or rash, depends largely on the pathogen and the viral/bacterial load within the bloodstream. Some infections have more profound consequences than others, including hospitalization. See appendix A for a list of infections that are relevant to the newborn period.

> Newborn infections generally present with one or more of the following signs: poor appetite, decreased activity, irritability, or an abnormal temperature (≤ 97.7°F or ≥ 99.5°F).

Establish healthy boundaries for visitors. Let's face it, newborns are a big deal, and nothing brings a family together like the birth of a baby! Grandparents are frequently anxious to spend time with the newest addition to the family. And while each family is different, the expectations surrounding this long-awaited arrival may be *unreasonably* high. On occasion, expectations are so high that visitation competes with the health and well-being of the mother or baby. My best advice is to establish healthy boundaries before bringing your newborn home from the hospital. Establish limits on the frequency and duration of visits, especially in the first days and weeks after delivery. Establish a schedule that makes sense for you and your newborn—not your visitors. An extra portion of grace may be needed for these conversations, but establishing healthy boundaries may be important to your baby's health and well-being, and perhaps your own! Soon enough, friends and family can come for longer, unscheduled visits.

Public exposures. When is it safe to take your newborn out in public—to church, the grocery store, or an outdoor event? The answer to this question is more difficult to accept for some than for others, especially for the sanguine personality. If you fall into this category, remember that newborns require more protection from the elements and infectious exposures than older children, and that the newborn period flies by! But this doesn't mean you need to be a hermit either. The vast majority of community-acquired infections are invisible to the human eye, so it is prudent to avoid public exposures until your newborn has established some physiologic resilience. In so doing, you will decrease the likelihood of a community-acquired infection and avoid the anxiety that accompanies such an infection. In a study published in 2019, nine percent of newborns with a viral respiratory illness were coinfected with a serious bacterial infection.[28] While most viral infections are self-limited and resolve without complication, the risks are greater in the first few months of life, and pediatricians are more likely to admit the *symptomatic* newborn to the hospital for observation and/or antibiotics.

My advice is to take a four-to-six-week stay-at-home vacation and to avoid public venues—to bond with your newborn, establish a routine, and balance the demands of your growing family. Skip the social scene for six weeks—both you and your baby will benefit! Later, when your newborn is thriving, cautious public exposures are less likely to pose a risk to your newborn's health and well-being. Infants born preterm (or small for gestational age) are at slightly greater risk than full-term infants. Therefore, depending on the gestational age, a slightly longer stay-at-home vacation

amniotic membranes is associated with amniotic fluid infection, which in turn is associated with preterm delivery and early-onset infection in the newborn.[61, 62] For this reason, the pediatric medical team must be careful to identify clinical risk factors after delivery, so appropriate steps can be taken.

On occasion, the umbilical cord becomes wrapped around the baby's neck (nuchal cord) during labor and delivery, compromising blood flow to the brain and vital organs. In extreme cases the cord can become knotted. Interruption of blood flow to the developing baby, for any reason, can result in fetal distress. In severe cases, the baby's heart rate decreases (decelerations), and the developing baby becomes compromised. If this occurs, an emergency delivery is needed to avoid brain damage (birth asphyxia). Each of these scenarios can complicate the care of an otherwise healthy pregnancy, which is why it is so important to have obstetrical and neonatal resuscitation teams available.

Unfortunately, fetal distress can result in passage of *meconium* into the amniotic fluid. Meconium is a collection of inspissated cells and secretions that slough from the intestinal walls during fetal development. It accumulates in the lumen of the intestines during pregnancy and passes from the rectum as the first several stools after delivery. Parents are often surprised to learn that meconium is sterile (noninfectious), but it is nonetheless noxious to the lungs, complicating roughly 10–15 percent of all deliveries. Meconium aspirated into the lungs and airways can cause a chemical pneumonia, otherwise known as *meconium aspiration syndrome*.[63] Thus, infants born through meconium-stained amniotic fluid may require suctioning of the mouth and airway at delivery.[64] If large amounts of meconium are aspirated into the lungs and airways, the lungs become so inflamed that oxygen and/or mechanical ventilation is needed. In such cases, the resuscitation team may insert an artificial airway (endotracheal tube) into the windpipe (trachea) to provide respiratory support. Fortunately, the majority of infants born through meconium-stained amniotic fluid require only minimal support. Close monitoring is important, however, as the signs of meconium aspiration syndrome can be delayed for minutes to hours after delivery.

The Initial Postpartum Assessment

Most babies are born at or near full-term gestation and require only minimal assistance with delivery. Immediately after delivery, an assessment of the newborn's gestational age, respiratory status, and neuromuscular tone is performed.[64] If any one of these is deemed abnormal, the newborn should be moved to a lighted radiant warmer for a more thorough examination and the initial steps of stabilization. The *initial steps* of newborn stabilization include warming, drying, and stimulating the newborn, and occasionally, clearing the mouth and airways of secretions.[65] A poor response to these initial steps suggests the need for additional supportive efforts. In some cases, oxygen or positive pressure ventilation may be needed to inflate the lungs or support spontaneous breathing. Usually, the need for additional respiratory support is transient and short-lived.

Fortunately, the vast majority of deliveries are uncomplicated.[66] Nonetheless, at least one person capable of providing newborn resuscitation must be present at every delivery.[64, 65] The Neonatal Resuscitation Program (NRP), in collaboration with the American Academy of Pediatrics and the American Heart Association, has established standards for newborn resuscitation, and most hospitals are eager to meet these standards of care.[66, 67] Birthing centers generally require their labor, delivery, and newborn staff to receive NRP training and certification.[65] Physicians, advanced practice providers, nurses, and respiratory therapists working in perinatal centers are typically expected to maintain this certification, which includes both cognitive and hands-on testing in the standards of neonatal resuscitation. Indeed, one of the most important reasons to deliver your baby in a hospital setting is to ensure that your newborn enjoys the benefits of this training and expertise.

The results of research on home births are mixed, but there is at least some evidence that home births are associated with a *slight* increase in the risk of newborn death.[68, 69] While I am a strong advocate for the use of midwives in prenatal and perinatal settings, I have a rather strong conviction that hospital births are safer than home births for both mother and baby. Hospitals have the equipment and personnel needed to deal with the complications that arise in the birthing process.

Delayed Cord Clamping

In recent years, labor and delivery units have become more holistic in their approach to delivery room care—and for good reason. One recent development is the adoption of delayed umbilical cord clamping. Delayed cord clamping, for as little as 30 seconds and as long as 3 minutes, has proven beneficial for term and late preterm newborns who are otherwise healthy.[70-72] This simple intervention increases the newborn's red blood cell concentration, resulting in an increase in the capacity of the bloodstream to transport oxygen to the tissues. The most common unintended side effect of delayed cord clamping is a slight increase in the risk of jaundice. This means that infants undergoing delayed cord clamping should have access to treatments for jaundice (e.g., phototherapy) and appropriate follow-up care with a pediatrician.[73] Therefore, if you live in a remote area without access to treatments for jaundice, delayed umbilical cord clamping carries a slightly increased risk of jaundice.

Skin-to-Skin Care

Skin-to-skin care is yet another example of a recent trend toward holistic newborn care. Skin-to-skin care is accomplished by placing the newborn on the mother's chest, skin-to-skin, just after delivery. Depending on the circumstances of the pregnancy and delivery, skin-to-skin care can be provided for as long as an hour. Assuming all the usual signs of well-being are present, skin-to-skin care allows mother and baby to bond, while simultaneously providing warmth and an opportunity to initiate early breastfeeding. Skin-to-skin care is now considered standard of care in most birthing centers in the US. In the absence of risk factors requiring intervention, infants who are at least 35 weeks gestational age, breathing comfortably, and both pink and warm to touch

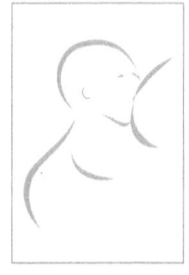

ID 47329083 © Fxmdk73 | Dreamstime.com

are good candidates for skin-to-skin care. The risk of respiratory and temperature instability is slightly greater for smaller, preterm babies, so infants born at less than 35 weeks *may not* be mature enough for skin-to-skin care. Most labor and delivery units have established standards for skin-to-skin care, and we will come back to this.

Skin-to-skin care enhances the success of breastfeeding and decreases the risk of infection in premature infants.[74, 75] Skin-to-skin care is also associated with physiologic stability and maternal attachment, reduced maternal anxiety, and enhanced newborn development.[76] And the same is true for infants with medical complications. In a study of infants with congenital heart disease, skin-to-skin care improved cognitive function and had a stabilizing effect on heart rate variability.[77] Skin-to-skin care is feasible after cesarean section, except when general anesthesia is required or when complications arise. In summary, research suggests that skin-to-skin care has benefits for both mother and baby and supports the important link between human touch and newborn brain development.

> Research suggests that skin-to-skin care has several benefits and supports my view that human touch is essential for healthy newborn brain development.

To summarize, the labor and delivery nurse or advanced practice provider will perform a *brief* assessment of the newborn's gestational age, breathing pattern, and muscle tone. This provides a general sense of the baby's overall health status just after delivery. If the initial assessment is concerning or even suspicious, the labor and delivery nurse (or practitioner) will perform a more thorough assessment of the newborn at a lighted radiant warmer or perhaps in a neighboring stabilization room. It follows, then, that at least one practitioner capable of providing newborn resuscitation should be present at each delivery.[65] If the initial assessment is reassuring, the newborn can be placed skin-to-skin for bonding and initiation of breastfeeding (if desired). Skin-to-skin care is generally allowed for at least 45 minutes, which is just enough time for mother-infant bonding and one breastfeeding attempt. This is among the most important evidence-based practices for promoting breastfeeding.[78]

The Newborn Physical Exam and Assessment

The postpartum newborn assessment is an evaluation of the newborn's overall health and well-being. In otherwise healthy newborns, it is performed by a nurse or advanced practice provider after an initial period of skin-to-skin care. It may be performed in the labor and delivery suite, where the mother is recovering, or in a well-lit room such as the newborn nursery. While each hospital has its own routine, the newborn assessment is followed by a careful review of the maternal record, so that potentially important risk factors can be identified. Any risk factors identified should be brought to the attention of the pediatric physician in a timely manner. Assuming no risk factors are identified, the labor and delivery nurse will facilitate mother-newborn bonding and healthy feeding patterns. If all the usual signs of well-being are present, the pediatrician's examination can wait until the following day. However, if risk factors are identified, diagnostic studies (e.g., laboratory studies) may be needed, even if the baby is well-appearing. The signs of illness are sometimes subtle in the newborn period, but the ill-appearing newborn should be evaluated by a physician or pediatric extender *without delay*.

Hospitals increasingly employ pediatric physicians who limit their practice to hospitalized infants and children. Some work exclusively in the newborn nursery setting, while others combine their outpatient (pediatric clinic) and inpatient (hospital) duties, maintaining hospital privileges that include newborn nursery coverage. Therefore, the physician or hospitalist caring for your newborn may (or may not) be affiliated with the pediatric group you have selected. If risk factors or clinical problems are identified during the assessment and review of maternal records, your pediatric physician will be contacted.

Preventive Measures

Eye care. Over the years, a number of public health initiatives have found their way into maternity units—and for good reason. The application of antimicrobial eye ointment (erythromycin) decreases the risk of *ophthalmia neonatorum,* an infection of the conjunctiva and orbit of the eye. *Ophthalmia neonatorum* is a vague term that describes a viral, bacterial, or chemical inflammation of the translucent membrane covering the white part of the eye (the conjunctiva). It generally occurs within the first month, and until the late nineteenth century was the leading cause of newborn blindness.[79] In 1881, Dr. Carl Franz Credé, a German obstetrician, introduced the use of silver nitrate as a strategy for preventing ophthalmia neonatorum.[79] A small ribbon of ointment applied to the lower eyelids at birth (after gently retracting the lower eyelids) resulted in a significant reduction in newborn eye infections.[80] The modern version of this strategy is the application of a single ribbon of erythromycin ointment to the lower lid of each eye just after birth. Admittedly, this preventive measure was established to prevent complications of sexually transmitted diseases. However, the treatment is so benign and so cost-effective that it has become the standard of care in most birth centers worldwide.

Vitamin K prophylaxis. Another important public health effort is the intramuscular administration of vitamin K, which decreases the risk of bleeding in newborns. Physicians now prefer the term *vitamin K deficiency bleeding*, as vitamin K deficiency is only one of several causes of bleeding in the newborn period. Vitamin K is important for blood clotting, and deficiency of this essential vitamin is associated with life-threatening bleeding in newborns. Vitamin K deficiency bleeding (from the mouth or gums, circumcision site, or intestinal tract) is rare in the modern era, in large part because of the widespread use of vitamin K. However, newborns are still at some risk for several reasons: (1) poor placental transfer of vitamin K (mother to baby) during pregnancy, (2) low levels of vitamin K in breastmilk, and (3) poor intestinal absorption of vitamin K.[81] The classic variant that occurs in the first week of life is easily prevented with a single low dose of vitamin K administered just after birth.[81, 82]

Umbilical cord care. Umbilical cord infection (omphalitis) is more common with home births, lotus births (where the umbilical cord is intentionally not separated from the placenta after birth), and births in developing countries.[83, 84] The high prevalence of omphalitis in the premodern era led to the use of *gentian violet*, a purple-colored medication with potent antimicrobial properties, which for many years was used in labor and delivery units to prevent this potentially life-threatening infection. However, in recent years gentian violet has gone out of favor due to its association with cancer development later in life. The current trend is to simply keep the umbilical cord clean and dry, at least until it dries up or falls off, which is usually within 10 to 14 days.[85] Alcohol swabs can be used to hasten drying of the cord, but this is generally unnecessary.[86] Omphalitis typically manifests as redness or swelling, a foul odor, or drainage of pus from the umbilical stump.[85] Additional cord care is appropriate for out-of-hospital births, lotus births, and births in resource-limited areas.

CHAPTER 5. THE TRANSITIONAL PERIOD AND DISCHARGE READINESS

The first hours of life are so important that they are sometimes referred to as the *golden hours*.[10] This transitional period begins with the first breath and is complete when the vital organs, especially the brain, lungs, liver, and adrenal glands, have fully adapted to postnatal life.[57] During pregnancy, oxygen intake, carbon dioxide elimination, and nutrient delivery to the developing baby are dependent on the interface of maternal and fetal blood within the uterus and placenta.[87] The lungs are fluid-filled, providing an important stimulus for lung development. During labor and delivery, lung fluid is expelled from the airways in preparation for breathing. With the clamping of the umbilical cord, oxygenated blood and nutrients are suddenly diverted to the newborn's lungs for oxygen uptake and subsequently to the heart for delivery to the tissues. Thus, after birth, delivery of blood and nutrients depends on the newborn's relatively immature lungs and circulatory system. Similarly, the regulation of temperature, blood pressure, blood sugar, and other vital functions are dependent on organs that are still undergoing adaptation to postnatal life.[88]

Despite the complexities of this important transition, most newborns are breathing spontaneously, pink in color, and warm to touch within minutes after birth. Most are capable of maintaining a normal core body temperature in an open crib and are able to participate in skin-to-skin care. Oral feeding reflexes are generally present but may not be fully mature on the first day. Nonetheless, with each feeding attempt, oral motor coordination and intake improves. Soon, the healthy newborn is arousing hungry every two to three hours and taking ever-increasing volumes of breastmilk (or formula). Feeding sessions are typically followed by a period of quiet contentment, and later by a period of sleep. Prematurity, low birth

43

weight, and retained lung fluid are among the most common factors to interfere with this normal physiologic transition, so these are addressed more completely in the chapters that follow.

> A newborn's arousal and interest in feeding is one of the most important signs of health and well-being.

Complications are rare, but when they occur, a qualified medical team is needed. Birthing hospitals that manage high-risk pregnancies generally have the staff and support systems to provide high-quality care. Likewise, hospitals that routinely care for complex newborn conditions, such as prematurity, respiratory distress, and birth defects, generally have the staff and support systems needed to provide optimal care.[89] If a high-risk delivery is anticipated, then obstetrical care and delivery in a high-risk birthing center is ideal. However, many families live in remote areas or near hospitals that lack these resources, so what is ideal may not be realistic. If maternal transfer to an appropriate facility is not safe or appropriate, then the best option becomes delivery in a community hospital, followed by stabilization and transfer of the newborn to an appropriate facility.[89] In either case, a well-organized delivery and stabilization plan, and communication with the high-risk perinatal center, will yield the best outcome.

Less than one percent of newborns require resuscitation in the delivery room—so it is a relatively rare event. Most infants are born between 39- and 41-weeks' gestation, without genetic abnormalities or malformations and without signs of illness or infection. While breast-fed newborns enjoy the benefits of passive immunity (maternal antibodies passing into the breastmilk), they are nonetheless vulnerable to viral and bacterial infections. Moreover, even healthy, full-term newborns can develop transient respiratory distress, difficulties with breastfeeding, or difficulties maintaining a normal temperature or blood sugar. For this reason, newborns should be monitored for a minimum of 24 hours after birth, preferably 36 hours, and some require up to 48 to 72 hours of observation before discharge is deemed safe and appropriate.

On the first day of life, or perhaps the following day, the pediatrician will review the obstetrical history and perform a thorough physical examination. Ideally, the nursery staff will have already identified important risk factors and notified the pediatrician. Together, your mother-baby nurse and pediatrician are charged with identifying infants in need of additional testing or monitoring. If risk factors are identified, your newborn's hospitalization may be prolonged, if only by a day or two, and the duration of the hospital stay depends on the nature of the risk factors identified, including poor feeding skills, weight gain/loss, and the presence or absence of jaundice.

A member of the pediatric team will perform a newborn assessment each day—generally in the morning—to determine whether hospital discharge is safe or appropriate. In the absence of risk factors, healthy newborns can be discharged as early as 24 hours after delivery. I am not a huge fan of early discharge, especially with first-time parents. However, if no risk factors are present and the baby is feeding, voiding, stooling, and maintaining a normal temperature in an open crib, then early discharge is reasonable. If jaundice, excessive weight loss, or poor feeding is noted, then your pediatrician may extend the hospital stay for another day (or two) depending on the circumstances of the pregnancy and delivery. Likewise, infants born preterm, including those born at 36 to 37 weeks' gestation, should be monitored until both mother and baby are ready for discharge. In some cases, early outpatient follow-up may be appropriate. The first follow-up visit (within two to three days) is generally brief, but important, and the pediatrician's primary objective is to ensure that the baby has all the usual signs of health and well-being and is thriving.

Discharge Readiness

For some, discharge readiness is a complete mystery, and concerns raised by the nursing staff or pediatrician are not always appreciated by parents! Keep in mind, however, that a delay in hospital discharge is generally for the *safety of the newborn*. While the criteria for a safe discharge varies from hospital to hospital and perhaps from pediatrician to pediatrician, the American Academy of Pediatrics has provided some helpful guidance: "The hospital stay should be long enough to identify problems unique to the pregnancy and delivery, and the mother should be sufficiently recovered and prepared to care for herself and her newborn at home."[(90)] I appreciate this guidance, as it is practical while recognizing two important concepts: (1) not all pregnancies and deliveries are the same, and (2) every discharge must be safe for both mother and baby.

A safe discharge. My interpretation of this guidance is that the length of stay should be based on: (1) the health of both mother and baby, (2) the ability and confidence of the mother to care for herself and her newborn, (3) the adequacy of support systems (father or significant other) at home, and (4) access to appropriate follow-up after discharge. Again, this guidance is practical because it emphasizes that each mother-baby pair is unique, with some needing more time (or support) than others. The late preterm infant, for example, may need an extra day (or two) to establish adequate nutritional intake or temperature control. Likewise, infants born by cesarean section, or those with social challenges, may need additional time for a safe discharge. Every mother-baby pair is unique and should be treated as such.

Adequate milk intake and weight gain. Several important signs of well-being should be documented before your newborn is deemed ready for discharge. The first and most important of these is adequate nutritional intake. If you haven't already, you will soon discover that this is a fundamental concept in the care of newborns, one we return to over and over again. Perhaps the single most important sign of well-being is the newborn's *appetite*. A newborn should arouse from sleep hungry every two to three hours around the clock. Moreover, the healthy newborn should ingest enough milk to regain his/her birth weight and sustain growth. Newborns may sleep as long as three to four hours on occasion, but healthy newborns should arouse with an appetite or hunger cues (rooting, turning toward the breast or nipple) on a regular, predictable schedule, generally every 2 to 3 hours.

Nutritional intake. Assessing milk intake is more challenging for breastfed newborns, especially in the first few days when the milk supply is limited. However, the observation of milk dribbling from the side of the mouth, audible swallowing, and a satisfied newborn are all signs of adequate intake. As the milk supply increases, nursing mothers also experience relief from breast engorgement after each feeding session. Voiding and stooling patterns provide additional evidence for adequate milk intake. Most newborns have one to two wet diapers on the first day, two to three on the second day, and three to six wet diapers on the third day. Thereafter, the healthy newborn generally has six to eight wet diapers per day. While subjective, each of these provides some evidence that nutritional intake is improving over time. Perhaps the most objective measure of adequate intake is weight gain, but even healthy newborns lose weight in the first few days, only to regain the weight lost within seven to ten days. For this reason, newborns are weighed daily in the hospital newborn nursery.

Anticipated weight loss. Newborns can lose as much as 5 to 7 percent of their birth weight in the first few days after birth.[91] The nursing team routinely monitors daily weights, as weight loss (and subsequent weight gain) is an objective measure of breastfeeding success and discharge readiness. A weight loss of 10 percent or more, for example, suggests that nutritional intake is inadequate for a safe discharge.[92] In such cases, supplementation with formula may be needed to achieve reversal of weight loss, if only for a few days. Excess weight loss is more common among exclusively breastfed newborns but is also seen after cesarean section (maternal stress). The good news is that most newborns achieve adequate intake within 72 hours. Reversal of weight loss typically follows the transition from colostrum to transitional breastmilk, but in rare cases can take as long as three to five days. The physiologic "let-down" provides evidence that mother's milk has come in, but a gentle stroke of the breast or nipple, the newborn's cry, and a good latch all promote milk production. Breast engorgement is yet another sign that the transitional milk has come in, and relief from the discomfort that accompanies breast engorgement is tangible evidence that the newborn has ingested breastmilk. Consultation with a certified lactation consultant can provide practical guidance and support for those experiencing delayed milk production. However, generous fluid intake, rest, and persistence are the most important ingredients for breastfeeding success.

Temperature stability. Another important test of discharge readiness is a newborn's ability to maintain a normal body temperature in an open crib. This is more relevant for late preterm infants and infants born small for gestational age, as the temperature control centers in the brain are less mature in these infants. However, even healthy, full-term newborns can develop cold stress in the first few days after birth—especially in a cold hospital room. Because temperature instability is one of several signs of acute illness in the newborn period, most pediatricians are reluctant to discharge a newborn who has had one or more episodes of temperature instability. Most require that temperature stability be documented for a predetermined period of time, perhaps 36 or 48 hours, before discharge is deemed safe and appropriate.

Voiding and stooling (the plumbing). Newborns are expected to void (urinate) within the first 24 hours of life and to pass at least one stool within 48 hours. There are several possible explanations for a newborn's failure to void or stool in a timely manner (all of them rare), but failure to accomplish these basic plumbing requirements suggests the need for additional diagnostic testing—either to ensure that the plumbing is in working order or to ensure the absence of an acute illness. Nutritional intake and clinical circumstances contribute to variable elimination patterns, but the healthy newborn should have several documented wet diapers and at least one or two stools before discharge. This standard also applies to newborns whose parents desire an early discharge (after only 24 hours of observation). I will not allow discharge of a newborn who has not voided (within 24 hours) or stooled at least once.

Jaundice. Newborns are routinely screened for jaundice, as the consequences of excessive jaundice can be serious. Red blood cells have a lifespan of about 120 days. As senescent red cells die off, their by-products are metabolized to *unconjugated bilirubin*, which at elevated levels (> 25 mg/dL) is toxic to the newborn brain. This toxic form of bilirubin is then metabolized (conjugated) by the liver to a less toxic form and eventually excreted by the body. Because the newborn liver is immature and unable to meet the metabolic demands of bilirubin metabolism, it accumulates in the bloodstream and manifests clinically as jaundice (yellow skin). The most severe forms of jaundice derive from maternal antibodies that cross the placenta and cross-react with red blood cells in the newborn's bloodstream. However, jaundice is also caused by breastmilk itself, which is believed to contain enzymes that increase bilirubin levels. Your pediatrician may prescribe *phototherapy*, which is a *light therapy in the blue-green spectrum* that metabolizes bilirubin to its nontoxic form. If phototherapy is needed, hospital discharge may be delayed until the bilirubin level is in a safe range.

Alternatively, close outpatient follow-up with bilirubin levels can be arranged after discharge.

Pre-discharge Screening Tests

Before discharge, the nursing staff will administer several screening tests designed to identify *potentially* dangerous congenital (present at birth) conditions. Three screening tests have become standard in most US hospitals and in many hospitals worldwide. The pulse oximetry screen identifies infants at risk for *critical congenital heart disease (CCHD)*, the state newborn screen identifies infants at risk for *inborn errors of metabolism,* and the universal hearing screen identifies infants at risk for *congenital hearing loss.* Each of these is based on evidence from the pediatric literature and, if negative, provides some assurance that the risk of these conditions is relatively low. Keep in mind, however, that newborn screening tests cannot rule out every possible adversity arising in the newborn period. *Screening tests* are low-cost tests designed to identify as many patients as possible with a given condition within the population. Like all screening tests, these newborn screening tests lack the *sensitivity* to identify every case in the population and lack the *specificity* to rule out all cases of the disease within the population. Accordingly, infants with a positive screening test should either be referred for evaluation by an appropriate specialist or receive a diagnostic evaluation *before* hospital discharge.

Screening test for critical congenital heart disease (CCHD). Congenital heart defects are categorized by the nature and severity of the defect. Whereas the vast majority of *congenital heart diseases* have excellent outcomes, the most serious defects are characterized as "critical" and carry a greater risk if diagnosis is delayed. Only eight out of every 1,000 live-born infants are diagnosed with a congenital heart defect, and less than 25 percent of these are deemed "critical" congenital heart defects. As such, the pulse oximetry CCHD screen is designed to identify a relatively small number of babies. Despite the complex nature of some of these conditions, survival for *critical* congenital heart disease continues to improve with advances in care.[93] Early identification is important, nonetheless, as a delayed or missed diagnosis increases the risk of a poor outcome.[94] Therefore, the CCHD screen is among the most important items on the discharge checklist.[95] It is performed no sooner than 24 hours after birth, and an abnormal (failed) screen warrants either an echocardiogram (ultrasound of the heart) or consultation with a pediatric cardiologist *before* hospital discharge.

The state newborn screen (NBS) for metabolic disorders. Metabolic disorders are rare, by comparison, with a worldwide prevalence of roughly one out of every 50,000 to 150,000 live births.[96] Otherwise known as *inborn errors of metabolism*, these disorders are abnormalities of the genetic pathways (within) the cells of the body. Unfortunately, some inborn errors are not amenable to treatment. In the last 10 to 15 years, however, technological advances such as tandem mass spectrometry have resulted in the development of expanded newborn screening (NBS) programs, which can identify more than 30 *potentially treatable* inborn errors—at a cost of less than $10 per newborn.[97] Early identification can be lifesaving, so metabolic screening programs are an important component of the public health system. The state newborn screen is obtained by collecting a few small drops of blood from a tiny heel prick just before discharge. A litmus-type paper/pad is saturated with the blood and then mailed to the state newborn screening laboratory for analysis. The results are generally available within two weeks—but this varies from state to state. Abnormalities are flagged and sent to the pediatrician designated at hospital discharge. Like many screening tests, the state newborn screen is unable to identify (or rule out) every possible disorder of metabolism.[97]

The universal hearing screen. Estimates vary widely, but the incidence of congenital hearing loss is approximately 1.9 cases per 1,000 live births in the US.[98] Because delayed diagnosis is associated with long-term language delays, early diagnosis is essential. Like other screening tests, the hearing screen (both otoacoustic emission and auditory brainstem tests) cannot identify every case of congenital hearing loss, and false positive tests do occur. However, early identification improves long-term language development, especially among those identified *early* in the first year.[99-101] Thus, the universal hearing screen is considered a standard of care in the US.[102] Infants with a failed screening test should be referred to an audiologist for definitive diagnostic testing and/or evaluation by an ear, nose, and throat specialist. False positive (failed) hearing screens are common, so it is important to remember that the hearing screen is just that, a "screening" test, and many infants who are referred for follow-up audiologic testing are determined to have normal hearing.

Mother-baby pearls. Finally, your nurse or pediatrician may identify items unique to *your* baby's care. Mother-baby nurses have a wealth of knowledge and experience, and many of the pearls I have acquired over the years were gleaned from seasoned mother-baby nurses. First-time parents should seize the opportunity to learn as much as possible from their nurse(s) before hospital discharge. Preterm infants have additional criteria for a safe discharge, including documentation of physiologic stability (temperature control, the absence of heart rate decelerations or oxygen desaturations) and satisfactory completion of a car seat test (test of physiologic stability while in a car seat). The car seat test is typically 90 minutes in duration, and a failed car seat evaluation suggests the newborn is not sufficiently mature for travel. Most pediatricians recommend an outpatient follow-up visit within two to three days of discharge or sooner, but the timing and specifics of follow-up are often unique to the newborn's needs.

Male circumcision. Many families choose to have their male newborns circumcised. While medically unnecessary, circumcision is common in many cultures, and the decision to circumcise is personal. Whatever your cultural or religious background, the decision is entirely yours, so your wishes should be respected by the healthcare team. Before performing a circumcision, your pediatrician (or obstetrician) will examine the penis carefully for signs of hypospadias (abnormal adhesions or abnormal development of the foreskin and penis). Circumcision should be avoided in infants with hypospadias, at least until the penis has been evaluated by a pediatric urologist. It is also important to monitor for bleeding in the first hour or so after the procedure, and the newborn should not be discharged if there is evidence of active bleeding. Circumcision is a benign procedure and requires minimal care, but gentle handling of the diaper area and the liberal use of petroleum jelly products can minimize discomfort. The circumcision site may be slightly red or inflamed for a few days, but infection is rare, and pediatricians typically examine the diaper area at the first follow-up visit.

CHAPTER 6. CONDITIONS ARISING AFTER DELIVERY THAT CAN DELAY HOSPITAL DISCHARGE

In this chapter we examine conditions encountered in the first few days after delivery and before hospital discharge. Each of the conditions that follow requires the attention of a pediatric physician, but *the good news is* that most are transient in nature and have excellent long-term outcomes. Many of these conditions are recognized within hours of birth, and some are so common that birthing centers have developed protocols to facilitate early detection and management. As with many conditions encountered in the newborn period, early recognition is important, which is why an entire chapter is devoted to the management of these transient, but generally benign conditions. If identified promptly and treated appropriately, infants with these conditions should have an excellent outcome.

Transient Respiratory Distress

In the final days of pregnancy, physiologic and hormonal events prepare the developing newborn for delivery and transition to postnatal life.[87] Clearance of fetal lung fluid in the third and final stage of labor plays a key role in preparing the newborn for breathing.[103] However, infants born precipitously, or those born by cesarean section, may retain fetal lung fluid, which may in turn lead to transient respiratory distress. *Tachypnea* is the term used by physicians to indicate rapid breathing, so your pediatrician may refer to this condition as *transient tachypnea of the newborn* (TTN).[104] By definition, then, this is a transient condition, manifesting as rapid breathing that typically lasts less than 48 to 72 hours. TTN is seen in roughly 1 percent of full-term infants and as many as 5 to 10 percent of preterm infants.[105] While oxygen saturation levels (the percentage of oxygen-saturated hemoglobin in the bloodstream) should be monitored, most newborns require little or no supplemental oxygen. However, since tachypnea is also a manifestation of other, more serious causes of respiratory distress, diagnostic tests, such as chest radiographs and blood tests, may be appropriate. Importantly, the causes of respiratory distress are sometimes unclear in the first hours after delivery, so close observation and precautionary antibiotics are appropriate until the diagnosis can be established.

Early-Onset Infection

Unfortunately, the risk of infection is greater in the newborn period than in any other period in the first year. Roughly 70 percent of bloodstream infections occur within the first three months; half of these occur in the first month, and the vast majority of these in the first week.[106] For this reason, screening to identify risk factors for early-onset infection has become the standard of care. As many as 25 percent of childbearing women are asymptomatic carriers (colonized) with group B streptococcus (GBS), the most common cause of early-onset bloodstream infection. Screening for GBS colonization is generally performed during prenatal visits between 34 and 37 weeks' gestation.[107, 108] If vaginal delivery is anticipated, GBS *positive* pregnancies are treated with prophylactic antibiotics to decrease the likelihood of infection within the first three days after birth. When combined with other risk factors, maternal GBS status allows the medical team to identify infants who are at greatest risk of early-onset infection with GBS.[107]

> Early-onset infection is a potentially avoidable complication of the early newborn period.

Approximately half of women colonized with GBS will transmit the bacteria to their newborns during labor. After amniotic membrane rupture, and in the absence of intrapartum prophylaxis with antibiotics, roughly 1–2 percent will develop early-onset GBS disease.[109] Due to the serious nature of the infection, GBS disease was deemed a significant public health threat. As a result, key stakeholders, including the American Academy of Pediatrics and the American College of Obstetricians and Gynecologists, worked diligently to identify cost-effective population-based strategies to reduce the risk of GBS infection. Since the institution of early prevention strategies in 1996, which were revised in 2002 and updated again in 2010, the rate of GBS infection has decreased from roughly two to three cases per 1,000 live births to less than 0.5 cases per 1,000.[107] This public health effort is viewed by most pediatricians as a huge lifesaving success. After almost 25 years of clinical practice, I have managed very few cases of GBS infection—far fewer than pediatricians in previous eras of care.

The risk of transmission is significantly lower among infants born by cesarean section, so antibiotics are reserved for women who are in active labor and anticipating a vaginal delivery. On occasion, labor progresses precipitously, and delivery occurs without sufficient time for prophylactic antibiotics (to decrease colonization). In these cases, the risk of GBS infection is slightly increased. Your pediatric medical team will consider these and other risk factors to determine whether laboratory screening tests are appropriate. Although full-term infants are more likely to acquire GBS infection, preterm infants are more likely to acquire an *E. coli* infection.[107, 108] Unfortunately, there is currently no proven strategy for prevention of *E. coli* transmission. Early recognition is imperative, as it increases the likelihood of a good outcome. So, one of the primary responsibilities of the medical team is to be alert for risk factors and clinical signs of infection in the early postnatal period.

> The immune system is functionally immature in the first days and weeks after birth.

Low Blood Sugar

Healthy newborns have several innate mechanisms for the prevention of low blood sugar levels during fasting states (between meals). For example, insulin levels generally decrease after birth and remain low for several days, thus decreasing the likelihood of low blood sugar levels. In addition, the fetal/newborn liver stores glucose in the form of glycogen, which then mobilizes glucose into the bloodstream when blood sugar levels are low.[110] Unfortunately, these normal responses can be altered or may be functionally immature in the early newborn (transitional) period.

Low blood sugar affects as many as 10 percent of all newborns but is most commonly encountered in infants that are either smaller or larger than expected.[110-112] Glycogen storage begins (in the liver) no sooner than 35 weeks' gestation. Therefore, infants born less than 35 weeks' gestation generally have inadequate glycogen stores for the mobilization of glucose stores during fasting states. Infants of diabetic mothers are exposed to excess glucose during pregnancy, which leads to elevated fetal blood sugar levels. The newborn pancreas produces insulin in proportion to the blood sugar level, which creates several problems. First, the combination of excess blood sugar and insulin act together as growth factors, resulting in excessive growth of the developing baby. Thus, infants of diabetic mothers are often born large for gestational age—so large, in fact, that some have difficulty passing through the birth canal (more on this later). Second, excess insulin production leads to dangerously low blood sugar levels after delivery, as insulin drives blood sugar out of the bloodstream and into the tissues.

Low blood sugar is concerning because even transiently low blood sugar levels are believed to have an impact on developmental outcomes. Glucose is the primary nutrient for brain cell function. So when blood sugar levels are low, the brain suffers.[110, 113, 114] Unfortunately, the long-term consequences of low blood sugar may be serious, including poor feeding and seizures.[30, 113-115] There is some controversy about the most appropriate threshold for treatment, but infants who are at risk for low blood sugar should receive a blood glucose screen soon after birth. If the blood sugar is low enough (i.e., less than 40 to 45 mg/dL), your pediatrician will initiate an appropriate treatment regimen, which may include oral glucose gel, supplemental formula feedings, or intravenous fluids containing glucose.[116]

Jaundice

Jaundice is a term used to describe the yellow/amber coloring of the skin (and eyes) in newborns with elevated bilirubin levels. Bilirubin is one of the by-products of red blood cells, which have a lifespan of only 120 days before being broken down into bilirubin. Unfortunately, elevated bilirubin levels are toxic to the brain. Jaundice is common in the newborn period because the liver is functionally immature and unable to keep pace with the load/demand for bilirubin metabolism. As the bilirubin level increases, the skin and the white part of the eyes (sclera) become increasingly yellow (jaundiced), starting with the head and face, working down to the trunk, and finally to the extremities. Several factors increase the likelihood of jaundice in newborns, but if the bilirubin accumulates to toxic levels (i.e., greater than 25 mg/dL), there is an increased risk of brain damage. For this reason, pediatricians are careful to monitor bilirubin levels in the early postnatal period and generally begin treatment if the level is high or increasing rapidly.[117]

All newborns are at some risk of jaundice, but depending on maternal and infant factors, some are at greater risk than others. One of the roles of your pediatric and nursing staff is to assess these risks soon after delivery and develop an appropriate plan. The most common causes of jaundice are breastmilk intake and mother/baby blood group incompatibility. Whereas breastmilk jaundice derives from the presence of enzymes in breastmilk, blood group incompatibility results from maternal antibodies passing into the newborn circulation (via the placenta), where they cross-react with newborn red blood cells. This cross-reaction results in the breakdown of newborn red blood cells, thus increasing the bilirubin concentration in the bloodstream. Occasionally, jaundice is related to excessive turnover of blood, as from bruising or birth trauma. If left untreated, the consequences of jaundice can be serious, but several treatment options are available. Most infants respond to phototherapy (i.e., light in the blue-green spectrum [430–490 nm]), which, when directed at the skin, metabolizes bilirubin to its nontoxic form. In extreme cases, jaundice requires admission to the neonatal intensive care unit (NICU), where more complex therapies and frequent monitoring are available.

Birth Trauma

Birth trauma is any injury that results from trauma during the birthing process. While only 2 to 3 percent of live births experience birth trauma, it is more common among infants born large for gestational age (LGA). LGA newborns are more likely to get "stuck" in the birth canal—usually at the head or shoulder (shoulder dystocia)—and may require either vacuum-assist (suction cups at the scalp) or forceps (metal calipers) maneuvers to facilitate extraction. Likewise, an abnormal presentation, such as a breech or transverse lie, is more likely to be accompanied by birth trauma. While these methods to extract the baby may seem barbaric, the challenge for the obstetrician is that prolonged delivery can lead to interruption of the blood supply to the newborn, which can result in brain injury (birth asphyxia).[118] One of the obstetrician's chief concerns is delivering a newborn without

> On occasion, traction is required to minimize the risk of brain injury, and this, in turn, can result in birth trauma.

brain injury. Whereas a fractured collarbone or arm or a superficial laceration to the scalp can heal in a matter of days to weeks, brain damage is *irreversible*! Therefore, birth trauma to the presenting parts is justified in order to minimize the risk of brain injury. So, if your baby is born with a broken collarbone or limb but remains neurologically intact, consider giving your obstetrician a big hug—he/she may have saved you a lifetime of heartache!

By now, it should be clear that the labor and delivery process can result in bumps and bruises to the scalp, limbs, and clavicles. Given the size of a newborn's head relative to that of the birth canal, it is surprising that birth trauma is not more common! The soft tissues of the scalp encounter significant shear stress during the final stages of labor, which often results in swelling, bruising, or hemorrhage within the scalp and soft tissues. The following conditions are related to soft tissues of the scalp and head, the clavicles and limbs, and to the nerves that innervate the arms and face, which are especially vulnerable to injury during vaginal delivery.

"Cone head" following a vaginal delivery. The most common pressure-related injury to the head and scalp is referred to by physicians as *caput succedaneum*. A benign, self-limited swelling of the scalp, "caput" is a generalized, boggy swelling of the presenting part of the scalp and occiput, which typically resolves without treatment within two to three days. Caput is so common, in fact, that it is a generally expected finding after a normal vaginal delivery. Superficial abrasions are also common, but treatment is

typically not needed. Infants with larger abrasions or lacerations can be treated, if needed, with topical ointments such as Bacitracin or Neosporin.

Cephalohematoma. Occasionally, pressure-related injury to the head results in hemorrhage within the superficial/outer layer of the *bones* of the skull. Less common than caput, this hemorrhagic collection of blood is referred to as a *cephalohematoma*. What distinguishes cephalohematoma from caput is that the swelling is limited to the affected bone(s) of the skull. Unlike caput, then, the swelling that accompanies cephalohematoma generally does not cross the midline soft spot (sagittal suture). Whereas caput presents as a boggy soft tissue swelling of the entire occiput/scalp, including the midline, cephalohematoma typically does not, unless there is both caput *and* cephalohematoma. Although caput resolves within a few days, cephalohematoma becomes hardened and resorbed by the body. Although resolution may take weeks to months, cephalohematoma is nonetheless a relatively benign condition.

Subgaleal hemorrhage. Perhaps the most serious birth injury or trauma to the head and scalp is referred to as *subgaleal hemorrhage*. Subgaleal hemorrhage is caused by traction and traumatic separation of the muscles of the scalp from their attachments at the cranial bones, resulting in bleeding within the soft tissue planes of the scalp and neck. Whereas caput and cephalohematoma are associated with relatively insignificant amounts of bleeding, subgaleal hemorrhage can result in significant blood loss. Fortunately, this is rare and usually resolves without treatment. Nonetheless, close observation is important with this type of scalp swelling, and serial laboratory testing (hemoglobin or hematocrit levels) is appropriate to ensure that blood loss is not excessive or severe. If significant blood loss is documented, observation in the NICU may be appropriate.

Clavicle fracture. Clavicle fractures are relatively common, especially after a vacuum-assisted or forceps delivery. Interestingly, roughly one out of every 250 live births is accompanied by a clavicle fracture.[119] While almost universally uncomplicated, clavicle fractures can be painful and may result in "splinting," or a painful grimace with handling. Infants that are irritable when picked up or when repositioned in the bassinette should undergo an evaluation for clavicle fracture, if only to confirm the diagnosis. Immobilization of the affected arm with baby blankets often minimizes the discomfort associated with handling. Virtually all newborns with a clavicle fracture recover with supportive treatment. Referral to an orthopedic surgeon should be reserved for the extremely *rare* case of a compound fracture (bone breaks through the skin) or a severely angulated fracture. In 25 years of clinical practice I have never referred a patient to an orthopedic surgeon for clavicle fracture.[119]

Brachial plexus palsy. Traction to the head and neck during delivery can result in transient weakness (palsy) of the nerves that innervate the shoulder, arm, and forearm.[120] The resulting injury, sometimes referred to as *Erb's palsy*, is caused by stretching or avulsion of the nerves that innervate the shoulder and biceps (proximal arm) during delivery/extraction of the newborn. Affected newborns are unable to rotate the shoulder and forearm or to raise the forearm from the table, but flexion of the fingers and wrist is usually preserved. The vast majority of brachial plexus injuries resolve without intervention within weeks to months.[121] Standard treatment includes immobilization of the affected arm/shoulder, referral to a physical or occupational therapist, and range of motion exercises. Infants who fail to regain full function within eight weeks should be referred to a pediatric neurosurgeon for possible surgical intervention—which is very rare.[120]

Unilateral facial palsy. Unilateral facial palsy resembles Bell's palsy, as it presents with a characteristic droop to one side of the face.[122] Less common than Erb's palsy, it is thought to be caused by stretching or bruising of a peripheral branch of the facial nerve. While forceps delivery is the most common association, the cause is not always apparent. This suggests that other traumatic mechanisms may be involved, including traction of the facial nerve during an otherwise normal delivery. Fortunately, most cases are transient, resolving within six months.[123] In one study, most infants with unilateral facial palsy were born without forceps, and the vast majority resolved within two months.[124, 125] Referral to a specialist (pediatric neurologist) is appropriate if the facial droop is still present at the four-month well-baby visit.

CHAPTER 7. CONDITIONS ENCOUNTERED IN THE NEWBORN PERIOD

Most pediatric office encounters involve benign, self-limited conditions. Caution is appropriate in the newborn period, however, as the signs of illness are often subtle, and delays in care can be consequential. Changes in appetite, activity, skin color, tone, or behavior suggest the possibility of an acute illness and should be brought to the attention of your pediatrician. In other words, the absence of the usual signs of well-being merits a prompt evaluation by a physician or practitioner. That being said, the vast majority of conditions encountered in the newborn period are benign and self-limited, so if the signs of health and well-being are present, you can generally be assured that your baby is fine. The aim of this chapter is to convey these concepts in the context of benign, uncomplicated conditions that are encountered frequently in the newborn period.

What Are the Signs of Health and Well-Being?

The ability to recognize the signs of health and well-being is fundamental to newborn care. However, as you get to know your newborn's sleeping and feeding habits, activity, and demeanor, recognizing deviations from these baseline characteristics becomes second nature. Changes in these characteristics or behaviors become so instinctive that the onset of illness is readily apparent to most mothers. For this reason, it is important to listen to your instincts and to seek medical attention when you have that feeling that "something's not right." Changes in appetite and demeanor are often among the earliest clues that something is wrong. Changes in skin color, tone, or activity, including lethargy or irritability, may come later but are certainly ominous, and provide additional evidence of the onset of an acute illness. Fortunately, the signs of health and well-being are relatively straight-forward.

When Should I Take My Baby in for a Doctor's Visit?

Childhood infections are often accompanied by the presence of a rash, but this is especially true of viral infections in the newborn period. While some infections are serious, many are not, and distinguishing those that are serious from those that are benign is nearly impossible in the outpatient (out-of-hospital) setting. Indeed, many infections that present with a rash are self-limited, so it is generally unnecessary to perform laboratory testing unless the newborn is ill enough to require hospital admission.

A useful question to ask is this: "Does my baby have all the usual signs of well-being?" A good appetite, normal temperature, normal

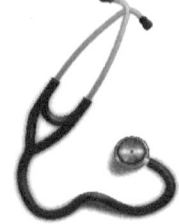

activity/behavior (level of alertness), and disposition? Does my baby arouse with signs of hunger every three to four hours, and is he/she able to keep meals down (without vomiting)? The first and most important of these signs, of course, is *appetite*. Poor appetite is among the

earliest signs of an acute illness, and since early recognition is important, a newborn's appetite is a critically important sign of health and well-being. Appetite is so important, in fact, that I often refer to it as the sixth vital sign. When evaluating infants (and young children) in the emergency department, the very first question I ask is this: "How is your baby's appetite?" Although it may be difficult to quantify feeding volumes in breastfed newborns, most nursing mothers are able to communicate if their newborn's appetite has changed.

The healthy newborn typically has a period of quiet contentment after meals, followed by a period of restful sleep. This, too, provides evidence that the newborn is ingesting sufficient quantities of breastmilk to be satisfied, to grow and to thrive. Skin color, temperature, and tone are also important, but changes in these clinical signs may appear later, and for this reason the characteristics of a rash, and other signs of well-being, are secondary in importance to a healthy appetite, disposition, and activity. Consider also that the presence of a healthy appetite and disposition can provide a great deal of reassurance. A newborn with a healthy appetite and disposition is generally a healthy newborn, and for this reason the answer to these questions is key to the evaluation of the potentially ill newborn!

The remainder of the chapter includes a brief summary of conditions that arise *after* hospital discharge. Infants who lack the usual signs of well-being should be evaluated by a pediatrician without delay, but the conditions that follow are generally accompanied by all (or most) of the signs of well-being. As such, these conditions are either benign or self-limited in nature and can be managed at home. Consider, however, that it is impossible in a short volume like this to include every possible benign, self-limited condition encountered in the newborn period. So the following is intentionally concise and intended to convey the principles or concepts of newborn health and well-being; it is not intended to be an exhaustive or comprehensive review of uncomplicated newborn conditions. If understood, however, these principles can be applied to an infinite number of circumstances, and should provide a common sense approach to conditions encountered frequently in weeks and months after birth.

Skin: Rashes, Skin Color, and the Signs of Well-Being

We begin with skin conditions because they are so common in early infancy and provoke so much anxiety among first-time parents. The rash that accompanies measles infection may be largely to blame for the level of anxiety created by newborn rashes, as measles has historical significance as a life-threatening viral infection. Consider, however, that most newborn skin conditions are benign or uncomplicated, and most can be monitored without treatment. While a rash may signify the presence of a viral infection, the most important determination is not the characteristics of the rash but the presence (or absence) of the signs of well-being, as already discussed. If, for example, a newborn has a fever, poor appetite, irritability, or lethargy, then regardless of the characteristics of the rash, a call (or visit) to your pediatric office or after-hours advice line is appropriate. In balance, while the characteristics of a rash are less important than other signs of well-being, the skin does provide some important clues regarding the newborn's health and well-being. And in some instances, the skin is a *window* through which one can determine the severity of a child's illness.

> While a rash may signify the presence of a viral infection, the most important determination is not the characteristics of the rash but the signs of health and well-being, as already discussed.

The skin is one of the newborn's first lines of defense against environmental hazards, including heat and cold, but especially against infection. But the skin also conveys important information about heart and lung function, and in this way, the skin provides a view of the newborn's overall health status. By controlling blood flow to and from the skin and extremities, the blood vessels of the skin and subcutaneous tissues play a key role in regulating temperature and blood pressure. In the healthy newborn, for example, the skin is warm and dry to touch and pink in color. Infants with poor (gray, mottled, or blue) skin color, or those with cool (poorly perfused) extremities should be evaluated by a physician without delay, especially when other signs of illness are present (fever, poor feeding, vomiting, etc.). This may be a sign of a heart or lung problem, or perhaps a life-threatening infection—any one of these requires the immediate attention of a skilled physician. On the other hand, the vast majority of skin conditions encountered in the newborn period are generally benign, resolving without treatment. Thus, recognizing the distinction between "normal" skin color and temperature (warm, pink, dry) and benign, self-limited rashes and skin conditions can be very helpful.

The following is a concise list of rashes, pigmented lesions, and vascular markings commonly encountered in otherwise healthy newborns. By definition, then, a newborn with any one of these conditions should have all the usual signs of well-being—a normal appetite, activity, disposition, and temperature (97.7°F to 99.7°F). While photos are not provided, many of the skin conditions discussed here can be found on the internet under the heading "newborn rashes." There are so many newborn rashes that a comprehensive review would defeat the purpose of this intentionally short handbook. Moreover, aside from the cutaneous signs of illness described in the previous paragraph, the characteristics of a rash are much less important than other signs of health and well-being.

Common, Self-Limited Skin Conditions

Acrocyanosis is a transient, blue discoloration (cyanosis) of the hands and feet (acro) that is most apparent just after birth. What distinguishes acrocyanosis from generalized or *central* cyanosis is that *acro*cyanosis is limited to the hands and feet, whereas central cyanosis is present at the central portions of the body, such as the anterior chest wall, lips, and tongue. Acrocyanosis results, in part, from constriction of the blood vessels in the extremities, and to some degree from the relatively high red blood cell concentration within the bloodstream just after delivery. Acrocyanosis typically resolves within several hours of birth but may persist for as long as 24 to 48 hours. As the transition from fetal to neonatal circulation progresses, the newborn's circulation improves and the palms and soles become pink. As such, acrocyanosis is a *transient phenomenon*, resolving soon after birth, whereas *central* cyanosis is generally associated with abnormalities of the heart and lungs or perhaps a bloodstream infection, any of which warrants a formal diagnostic evaluation by a pediatric physician.

Mottling of the skin. Mottling of the skin is characterized by patchy areas of pallor and red-to-purple marbling of the skin. Unfortunately, mottling can be seen in both healthy and sick newborns. It is most commonly seen in healthy newborns in cool environments. Mottling is often seen after removing a newborn from a warm bath in a cool room or when transitioning from warm to cool environments. Under normal circumstances, mottling resolves quickly after bundling or on return of the newborn to a warm environment. Mottling is the body's attempt to restrict blood flow to the skin and peripheral tissues—either to retain heat or to maintain blood pressure and perfusion to vital organs. Therefore, mottling can *also* be a sign of either a bloodstream infection or cardiovascular collapse (shock), but only in the context of other signs of acute illness—poor feeding, irritability, lethargy, or fever. Mottling that fails to improve with rewarming or bundling should prompt a careful evaluation for illness. Moreover, mottling that is observed in the context of other signs of illness should be brought to the attention of your pediatrician immediately. In the presence of all the usual signs of well-being, however, simply returning the baby to a warm environment should reverse the process and result in the return to normal skin color and perfusion.

Mongolian spot. Perhaps the most common *pigmented* birthmark in the newborn period is the Mongolian spot. Typically seen in the region of the lower back and buttocks, Mongolian spots are blue-gray in color and more common in African American, Asian, and Hispanic populations.[126] Mongolian spots derive from dense collections of melanocytes, the cells of the skin that produce pigment, and are generally *not* associated with other birth defects or anomalies.[126] More prominent at birth, mongolian spots typically disappear within one to two years. It is a benign discoloration, so referral to a specialist is unnecessary.

Stork bite marks. A stork bite mark is a pink to purple discoloration of the skin, most frequently seen on the brow of the face, head, or neck. Also known as a *salmon patch*, this vascular marking results from engorgement or stretching of the blood vessels within the affected area of skin. The salmon patch can be seen at the bridge of the nose or brow, the upper lip, eyelids, forehead, or at the nape of the neck. It is a transient phenomenon that fades within two to three months of birth. Seen in roughly one-third of all live births, it is among the most common vascular anomalies of the newborn period.[126] Once again, treatment is unnecessary, and the most prominent salmon patches will resolve within 12 to 18 months of birth.

Erythema toxicum. The term *rash* is typically reserved for *transient* vascular abnormalities of the skin. One of the most common rashes of the newborn period is *erythema toxicum*. Roughly one out of every five newborns develops erythema toxicum within the first few days after birth, frequently before leaving the hospital.[126] The name describes the rash well, as it is both red (erythematous) and toxic (toxicum) in appearance.[127] However, despite the inference, the rash is neither toxic nor dangerous, so its presence should not provoke concern. It typically presents as tiny red bumps (papules) surrounded by a red halo and is often found in crops that migrate from one region of the trunk/body to another. Erythema toxicum is benign and resolves without treatment within two to three weeks, never to be seen again.

Transient neonatal pustular melanosis. Less common than erythema toxicum, transient neonatal pustular melanosis is yet another uncomplicated, self-limited rash of the newborn period. It is characterized by multiple tiny pustules (tiny, pus-filled bumps) that evolve over days to weeks.[127] What starts as tiny pustules is later replaced by small, flat pigmented dots resembling freckles that disappear without a trace. As with erythema toxicum, neonatal pustular melanosis is benign and resolves without treatment or consequence.

Benign cephalic pustulosis. Benign cephalic pustulosis is another benign skin condition that affects as many as 60 percent of all newborns at one time or another.[127] Like other newborn skin conditions, it is self-limited and characterized by multiple tiny papules (bumps) and pustules (fluid-filled bumps), primarily on the face and scalp. It typically presents within the first month of life and is considered by many to be a neonatal variant of acne. As the name implies, it is both benign and inconsequential, resolving almost as soon as it appears.

Milia. Also known as *milia rubra,* milia is a red, slightly raised punctate rash that is common to the newborn period. Milia rubra results from obstruction of the sweat glands in the outer layer of the skin (epidermis). Sometimes referred to as *prickly heat*, milia is seen in as many as 16 percent of live births.[126] It is frequently seen in warm, humid environments, especially during the summer months, or in temperate climates. Like other rashes encountered in the newborn period, milia rubra is benign and transient. Removing the baby from the warm, humid environment, providing clothing that breathes well (such as thin cotton clothing), or simply turning on the central air-conditioning will result in improvement over time.

Atopic dermatitis. *Atopy* is a term that describes an individual's predisposition to allergies. Thus, *atopic dermatitis*, otherwise known as eczema, is an allergic condition of the skin. It typically manifests as patches of dry skin with tiny papules and a coarse texture resembling sandpaper. Atopic dermatitis is often a localized reaction to topical allergens, such as soaps or chemicals. However, when seen over the entire body, eczema may signify a systemic allergic exposure, such as allergy to cow's milk protein, which is found in commercial formulas. Avoiding the offending agent is usually adequate, but the use of mild soaps, such as Dove or Tone, and fragrance-free lotions, such as Cetaphil or Eucerin, is also helpful. Cotton clothing is preferred over synthetic fabrics, as synthetic materials are more allergenic. Severe allergic dermatitis may require a short course of topical steroids (e.g., 0.5% to 1% hydrocortisone for 5 to 7 days) and/or referral to a dermatologist. In extreme cases a stepwise plan to eliminate potential offending agents may be needed.

Contact dermatitis. One of the most common skin conditions encountered in newborns is contact dermatitis. Contact dermatitis is essentially an irritation of the skin resulting from *contact* or topical exposure to an irritant, whether it be a chemical, soap, synthetic material, or, you guessed it, urine and stool, which are the most common offending agents! Typically, the reaction occurs at the site of exposure, and the longer the exposure, the more severe the reaction. Unfortunately, contact dermatitis closely resembles a localized allergic reaction. However, the reaction to soaps, fragrances, and chemical irritants is typically "angrier," or red, and is often painful, which is different from eczema (dry, scaly, and associated with itching). Elimination of potential irritants, one by one, is the most appropriate initial approach. Low-potency topical corticosteroids (0.5% hydrocortisone) can provide relief, but barrier creams and petroleum-based creams and emollients (CeraVe' and Eucerin) are appropriate—especially for severe diaper rashes.

Candida (yeast) skin infections. Candida dermatitis, sometimes referred to as a yeast infection, is also relatively common. Yeast infections are sometimes difficult to distinguish from *contact dermatitis*, as both conditions present with a red, inflamed base and are accompanied by small, raised (papular) lesions or bumps. The one feature that distinguishes candida dermatitis from contact dermatitis is the location of the rash—candida is more commonly found in moist environments, like the inguinal creases and skin folds within the diaper area. Unfortunately, the diaper area of most newborns is universally moist, so yeast infections are seen in both the skin folds and exposed areas. Exposure to antibiotics increases the risk of a yeast infection, as antibiotics affect the balance of the intestinal microbiome, allowing for overgrowth of yeast. The initial treatment for a yeast infection is nystatin—powder for the moist skin folds and cream for the exposed areas.

Oral candidiasis. Newborns are also prone to develop candida (yeast) infections on the mucosal surfaces within the mouth. Also known as *oral thrush*, yeast infections in the mouth are characterized by white patches or plaques on the tongue and sides of the mouth, which are typically difficult to scrape off with a tongue depressor. Oral thrush is a relatively benign condition, but it can affect oral feeding skills, if only transiently. For this reason, treatment is appropriate, and the most appropriate first-line treatment is oral nystatin suspension, which requires a physician's prescription. Unfortunately, oral thrush is sometimes resistant to nystatin, so more potent prescription medications are sometimes needed. Overall, infants with oral thrush should have most of the usual signs of well-being, with the one important exception being a slightly diminished interest in feeding.

Keratin pearls. Keratin pearls are seen exclusively on the roof of the mouth. These tiny white "pearly" bumps are found on the hard and soft palate of the newborn's mouth. A benign condition that resolves without treatment, these small white bumps are essentially small inclusion cysts of keratin (skin/mucosal cells).

Common Gastrointestinal Conditions

Gastroesophageal reflux. Gastroesophageal reflux (i.e., GER or reflux), is one of the most common conditions encountered in the newborn period, experienced by as many as 75 percent of newborns in the first two months of life.[128] Most cases are asymptomatic, resolving without treatment within four to six months.[128] Asymptomatic infants are often referred to as "happy spitters," as there is no pain or discomfort and no clinical side effects.[128] Several factors increase the likelihood of GER in newborns, including a universally liquid-based diet, recumbent (flat) positioning, and weakness of the muscles of the lower esophagus.[129] Asymptomatic newborns with evidence of good weight gain should be monitored conservatively, but simply decreasing the duration of breastfeeding attempts (or the volume of formula offered) and increasing the frequency of meals can decrease the frequency and severity of reflux events. Additionally, keeping the baby slightly elevated for 15 to 20 minutes after meals can lessen the frequency and severity of events.

An occasional cough or choking spell is common, and most healthy newborns have airway protective reflexes that minimize the risk of aspiration of milk into the lungs. On the other hand, infants with persistent vomiting, poor weight gain (failure to thrive), or irritability (grimacing, arching after feeds) meet criteria for *symptomatic GER*.[128] Symptomatic GER is referred to as gastroesophageal reflux *disease* (GERD), which may also present with a chronic cough. In extreme cases, intermittent airway obstruction is observed, which may be accompanied by changes in skin color and/or wheezing. Reflux events associated with acute changes in breathing or skin color should be evaluated by a pediatrician. Experienced pediatricians typically have a stepwise approach to diagnosis and management of symptomatic GERD. Most pediatricians start with a trial of small, frequent feedings and elevation (for 15 to 20 minutes) after meals. GER that persists or is associated with irritability, arching/gagging, coughing/wheezing, or failure to thrive deserves consideration of a trial of medication. Famotidine is a safe first-line medication, but a stepwise elimination of potential offenders such as cow's milk protein should also be considered.

The complexities of reflux management illustrate the benefit of establishing a partnership with a seasoned pediatrician. Symptomatic reflux warrants further investigation, and most experienced pediatricians can do this with their eyes closed. Treatment options include medications that either block the effects of stomach acid, such as famotidine, or decrease the production of acid (proton pump inhibitors), such as omeprazole, esomeprazole, and lansoprazole. Ranitidine was previously available as an acid blocker but was removed from the market due to concerns about potential side effects. Famotidine has similar acid-blocking properties but without known side effects. When appropriate, these medications decrease the discomfort associated with reflux events, and improvement is usually noted within seven to ten days.[130]

Cow's milk intolerance/allergy. The terms *cow's milk allergy* and *cow's milk intolerance* are used interchangeably and refer to an intolerance (allergy) to the *protein* component in commercial cow's milk formulas. Cow's milk allergy is among the most common causes of symptomatic GERD in the first year of life.[131] Symptoms vary from mild intolerance (excessive gas, frequent stooling) to frank intolerance, with bloody, mucus-filled, watery stools, eczema, and poor weight gain (failure to thrive). The observation of blood or mucus in the stool is not required for the diagnosis, but severe cases are generally accompanied by one or more of these signs. In theory, sensitivity to cow's milk develops over time, after repeated exposures to cow's milk protein. Although cow's milk intolerance is by definition a sensitivity to the *protein* component in milk, not the carbohydrate (sugar) component, lactose-reduced formulas may provide some benefit.[132] Mild, *relatively* asymptomatic milk intolerance is more common, of course, so when treated promptly, severe disease can be avoided.

The signs of milk protein intolerance are observed in as many as 5 to 15 percent of newborns in the first two months.[131] However, as few as 3 percent of newborns are diagnosed, and less than 1 percent of breastfed newborns are symptomatic.[131-134] There is no single laboratory test for the diagnosis of cow's milk sensitivity, so diagnosis is typically established by obtaining a clinical history and by elimination of cow's milk from the diet.[135] Most affected infants are symptomatic by one month of age, and roughly half of these develop dry scaly skin (eczema) or gastrointestinal signs. The principal treatment is avoidance of cow's milk protein, but clinical improvement can take as long as one to three weeks.

Less than 20 percent of the infants diagnosed with cow's milk intolerance are also allergic to soy-based milk protein formulas.[136, 137] Some infants with cow's milk intolerance tolerate soy-based formula, but many will eventually require hydrolyzed (proteins are broken down) cow's milk formula. Hydrolyzed formulas, such as Nutramigen, Pregestamil, and Alimentum, are easier to digest and are found in most grocery stores. In extreme cases, an *elemental* formula (Elecare, Neocate) may be needed, but this is rare. Elemental formulas require a physician's prescription and are extremely expensive, so they are generally reserved for infants with severe disease (i.e., bloody stools, failure to thrive) or those who remain scoops of most 20 kcal/oz formulas can be mixed with 3.5 oz (105 mL) of water to yield a 22 kcal/oz formula. If needed, the additional calories and nutrients provide the calcium, phosphorus, and protein needed for catch-up growth. Importantly, however, fortification of breastmilk or formula should be directed by an experienced nurse, dietitian, or physician, as mixing errors have been known to result in dangerously high sodium levels and in some cases seizures.[31]

Formula-fed infants. Newborns fed with commercially available cow's milk formula may take as little as 5 to 10 mL (5 mL = 1 teaspoon) during initial feeding attempts. However, feeding volumes typically increase with each subsequent feeding and each subsequent day. Most newborns will take much as 30 to 45 mL (30 mL = 1 ounce) per feeding before hospital discharge. As with the breastfed newborn, excessive weight loss is a sign of inadequate intake, and reversal of this trend should be documented before hospital discharge.

Breastfeeding: Benefits and Challenges

Breastfeeding is one of the most positive things you can do for your baby! It is not easy, and it is not for everyone, but the rewards are substantial. To begin, breastfeeding creates an opportunity for bonding with your baby, which has been shown to have significant social, emotional, and developmental benefits.[32] Breastmilk provides immune protection and growth factors that stimulate normal growth and brain development.[33] Breastfed children have a lower incidence of infectious diseases, obesity, and metabolic disorders, as well as slightly better cognitive outcomes, than infants fed commercially available cow's milk formulas.[33] Lactose, the carbohydrate (milk sugar) component, constitutes the largest component of human milk. The protein is largely casein, but lactalbumin, lactoferrin, immunoglobulin A, lysozyme, and albumin are also found in breastmilk.[34]

The smaller components vary from mother to mother but include a number of important vitamins. The immune protection conferred by breastmilk derives largely from immunoglobulin A (IgA), which provides protection at the surface of the intestines, and lactoferrin, which limits the availability of iron to bacteria.[35] The point here is that science and evidence strongly support the benefits of breastmilk over cow's milk for newborn growth and development.

Breastmilk has benefits far beyond those attributed to nutrition and immune defense. Vascular endothelial growth factor and epidermal growth factor, which are widely known for their benefits in tissue growth and repair, are frequently found in breastmilk.[34] Likewise, insulin-like growth factor and brain-derived neurotrophic factor stimulate both brain growth and development. These growth factors and hormones are unique to breastmilk and not found in cow's milk formulas. Thus, breastfeeding provides tangible, long-term benefits for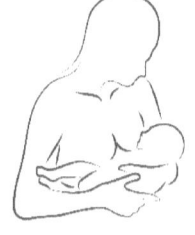

by mcmurryjulie via Pixabay

your newborn's health, well-being, and development, and the advantages of breastmilk over commercially available formulas cannot be overstated.

At the end of the day, however, breastfeeding is not for everyone, and sometimes the reasons are personal. So, whatever your reasons, your nutritional choice for your newborn should be respected and supported by the healthcare team. For those who work outside the home and wish to continue breastfeeding after parental leave has expired, the storage of breastmilk becomes a concern. The "rule of fours" is a simple yet helpful rule that applies to the storage and use of expressed breastmilk. *Breastmilk can remain in the freezer for as long as four months, in the refrigerator for as long as four days, and on the counter (outside the refrigerator) for as long as four hours.* Therefore, when pumping or manual expression of breastmilk is anticipated, some planning is required, and the *rule of fours* provides practical guidance on how to do this safely. Labeling milk bottles or canisters with dates and times and developing a storage system that works for you and your family (or your refrigerator and freezer) are important practical matters to consider up front.

> Rule of fours: breastmilk can be safely stored in the freezer for as long as four months, in the refrigerator for as long as four days, and on a countertop for as long as four hours.

Breastfeeding and newborn brain development. Breastfeeding provides important developmental benefits, including those related to human touch.[21] Brain development begins early in pregnancy and depends on the net sum of exposures and experiences encountered early in life. Early in gestation, nerve cells are born deep in the mid-brain—migrating to the outer mantle (cortex) of the brain by the end of the second trimester. Growth factors and hormones unique to breastmilk are believed to have a significant role in this process. Importantly, both sensory and environmental exposures have been shown to affect brain development during these formative weeks and months. As such, skin-to-skin bonding, which facilitates breastmilk production and breastfeeding success, are aspects of human touch that provide positive, developmentally appropriate stimulation for the developing brain.

Breastfeeding and vitamin supplementation. While breastmilk has numerous advantages, it is believed to be deficient in a few key nutrients, especially vitamins K and D. Vitamin K is essential for blood clotting, and for this reason, a single dose (0.5 mg intramuscular injection) has become the standard of care for many industrialized nations, including the US. Breastmilk is also deficient in vitamin D, which is essential for bone mineralization.[36] Maternal vitamin D deficiency is common in several ethnic populations, and when present can have adverse effects on the newborn.[37] Breastfed newborns are at slightly greater risk of vitamin D deficiency, so dietitians recommend that newborns receive 400 international units (IU) of vitamin D per day.[38, 39] Vitamin D is usually packaged as cholecalciferol (vitamin D_3) in concentrations of 400 international units/milliliter (IU/mL), so the recommended volume for a full-term breastfed newborn is one mL per day. Because formula-fed infants receive some (but not all) of the needed vitamin D in commercially available formulas, only 200 IU of vitamin D is recommended for formula-fed babies, until the *total formula intake* is at least 34 ounces (1 liter) per day.[39]

Breastfeeding Technique

Let's face it; some aspects of breastfeeding are simply *not* intuitive, and placement of the infant on the breast is one example of this. The newborn's mouth and lips should be positioned at the inferior margins of the areola, so that the mouth and lips are *widely opened, covering both the nipple and a sizable portion of the areola.* This positions the tongue for displacement of the areola *and* nipple toward the roof of the newborn's mouth (palate) for optimal milk expression. Placement of the mouth over the nipple *alone* can lead to pain or discomfort, inefficient feeding, and inadequate milk intake. Obstruction of the baby's nostrils (with breast tissue) can interfere with breathing, so it is important to monitor the placement of your newborn on the

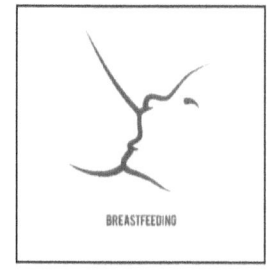

BREASTFEEDING

ID 53908215 © Chelovector | Dreamstime.com

breast during feeding sessions. Images and diagrams are available on the internet under the heading "good latch pictures." These websites are helpful and provide illustrations for positions such as the *cradle hold*, the *football position*, and the *side-lying position*. Each has its own merits, so an individualized approach is needed. In one study, breastfeeding in the *side-lying* position minimized maternal fatigue, and secondhand reports from nursing mothers, nurses, and lactation specialists support this conclusion.[40]

reaches for toys, rolls from back to front, and can elevate to the forearms/elbows when placed face down on a flat surface. A six-month-old is increasingly social, responds when called by name, brings hands and fingers to mouth, passes toys from hand to hand, and sits briefly without assistance. It is important to draw on your pediatrician's experience before getting too worried about minor deviations, as these are often explained by differences in the home and social environment. A tincture of time is generally all that is needed for age-appropriate milestones to emerge.

Neurologic status. An experienced pediatrician is generally able to assess an infant's neurologic status from across the room. A newborn's posture, for example, is often the first thing a pediatrician will notice when entering the examination room. Does the newborn make eye contact, coo, smile, or turn to voice? These observations can provide insight into a newborn's vision and hearing and can be made before laying hands on the baby. Likewise, a newborn's spontaneous activity and responses to stimulation during the exam are helpful. When combined, these observations provide a general impression of the newborn's developmental status. The physical exam often supports these observations but is nonetheless important. For this reason, it is my conviction that telehealth visits should not replace the physical examination. Muscle mass, neuromuscular tone (response to passive range of motion), and primitive reflexes, all of which evolve in the first year, are important aspects of the neurologic exam, and none of these can be adequately assessed via video or telehealth.

Vision. Newborns generally have lower visual acuity than older children and adults. In addition, the newborn's eyes may move disconjugately (they do not work together), which can be troubling to first-time parents. Rest assured, however, that this is completely normal in the first few weeks after birth. If disconjugate gaze persists beyond two to three months, a pediatric ophthalmologist should be consulted. By four to six weeks of age, a newborn should regard the face, especially that of Mom and Dad. Most newborns focus on objects within eight to twelve inches of the face, so it is important to get close in the first few days and weeks after birth. Contrasting colors and shades, especially red, black, and white, are appropriate for stimulating the vision centers in the brain and are a worthwhile investment in your newborn's early development. Roving eye movements are common, especially when the baby is sleepy or fatigued. The eyes may even appear to "roll back" (toward the top of the head) when emerging from sleep. With time, eye development progresses, and hand-eye coordination begins to emerge. Infants can usually track objects that are passed in front of them by two to three months of age, which generally corresponds to emergence of a social smile—an exciting development!

Hearing. Hearing is fundamentally important to early newborn development and highly related to language development later in life. Therefore, it has become standard of care in most hospitals to screen for congenital hearing loss before discharge. Given the importance of hearing to newborn development, a failed or "referred" hearing screen should prompt the mother-baby or newborn nursery staff to provide a referral to an audiologist within four to six weeks of hospital discharge. Many patients referred for hearing evaluation will subsequently "pass" either an otoacoustic emission (OAE) or auditory brainstem response (ABR)—the two most common tests of hearing for newborns. Further, most infants referred for audiologic testing are found to have *normal* hearing after audiologic testing has been completed.[51] Follow-up with an audiologist (or ear, nose, and throat physician) is important, nonetheless.

Posture and tone. Posture and tone are important characteristics of a neurologically healthy baby and important signs of newborn well-being.[52] Posture and tone also tend to parallel other signs of well-being, such as the newborn's vital signs, appetite, and activity. In this way, posture and tone are fundamental to the newborn physical exam. *Posture* is the position of the newborn's extremities relative to the trunk or torso (midsection of the body), especially when lying on a flat surface and undisturbed. While lying flat on a firm mattress, a *normal newborn* will rest with arms and forearms in a position of *slight flexion* across the torso, with the hands adducted toward the midline. In fact, the observation of the newborn's arms and hands at (or near) the midline is an important sign of neurologic health—one that I look for regularly in clinical practice.

Neuromuscular tone relates to a newborn's response to *passive range of motion* of the upper and lower extremities—especially at the hips, knees, and ankles but also at the shoulders and elbows. The healthy newborn generally has mild to moderate resistance to passive range of motion at the elbows, hips and knees. While this assessment is subjective, and best performed by 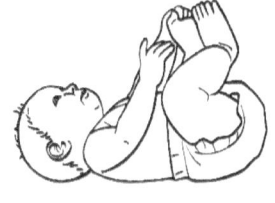 *by Clker-Free-Vector-Images via Pixabay* an experienced physician, abnormalities of tone are uncommon. When present, the experienced pediatrician will easily recognize abnormal neuromuscular tone. Acute/transient changes in neuromuscular tone are more common, especially among infants with an acute illness or infection. If persistent, however, abnormal tone should prompt a search for more serious causes. Newborns with minimal resistance to passive range of motion, or those with progressive worsening of neuromuscular tone, are said to have *hypotonia*, whereas those with increased tone are said to have *hypertonia*. It is worth noting, however, that over the course of the first year of life, neuromuscular tone gradually decreases—a normal developmental process.[53]

> Any concerns you may have about your newborn's posture or tone should be brought to the attention of your pediatrician.

Finally, visual, auditory, and language stimulation are all fundamental to newborn development. Talking and singing to your baby, making eye contact, and smiling at your baby are important means of stimulating the visual and auditory centers in the brain. Skin-to-skin contact is important as well, especially in the first weeks and months after birth. As already discussed, research supports a significant relationship between human touch and newborn brain development. Newborns appreciate being bundled with a blanket, as blankets provide warmth, minimize radiant heat loss, and provide boundaries that simulate being held by Mom and Dad. However, no amount of bundling can impact your baby's development like skin-to-skin touch and face-to-face interaction. The use of blankets should be discontinued at about two months because of the increased risk of accidental suffocation during sleep. We will address the topic of safe sleep in more detail in a later chapter.

CHAPTER 4. PREGNANCY, LABOR & DELIVERY, AND EARLY POSTNATAL CARE

Newborns are uniquely vulnerable in the first month of life, as immature organ systems undergo adaptation to postnatal life.[54-56] The newborn is especially vulnerable in the first postnatal week, as vital organs such as the heart, lungs, and brain undergo a rather sudden *transition* from intrauterine life, in which the physiologic demands of life are met almost entirely by the mother, to newborn life, in which the demands of life are met by the newborn's relatively immature organ systems. This means that newborns require special care and attention in these first days and weeks after birth.

During gestation, oxygen and nutrients are transferred from the mother to the developing baby by way of the placenta and umbilical cord. Anything that affects the development, attachment, or function of the placenta and uterus can result in poor growth, preterm delivery, or unexpected bleeding.[57] This is why routine prenatal care is so important. Obstetricians monitor the pregnancy by periodically checking the growth of the developing baby, amniotic fluid volumes, umbilical

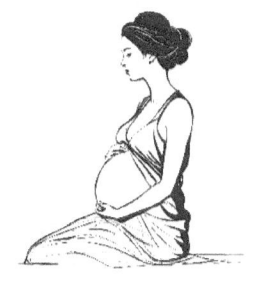

by ArturGórecki via Pixabay

cord blood flow, and placental attachment, among other things. Abnormalities detected during prenatal screening visits may alter the course of the pregnancy—for example, by necessitating preterm induction of labor and/or delivery by emergency cesarean section. If preterm delivery is recommended, then the obstetrician has presumably identified one or more risk factors for an adverse outcome for the mother, the baby, or both. The ethical dilemma this presents is complex, but most obstetricians consider the health and well-being of the mother a priority, as the mother has a central role in the life of the family.

Complications of Pregnancy

First, the complications of pregnancy are included here, if only briefly, due to their impact on both the delivery and the newborn's transition to postnatal life. Pregnancy complications arise with some regularity. In a study of over 300,000 pregnancies in the US, roughly 47 percent had at least one complication requiring medical decision-making.[58] Thus, it is my strong opinion that the birth of a newborn should occur in a birthing center, where obstetrical support is available twenty-four hours per day, seven days per week. Second, pregnancy complications can have adverse effects on both the mother and developing baby, and it is imperative for newborns to have an appropriate support team, when needed. Depending on the nature of the problem, the timing, mode of delivery (vaginal or cesarean section), or outcome of the pregnancy may be affected. Although I am a strong advocate for midwifery, I am an even stronger advocate for hospital deliveries, as delivery in a hospital setting provides a safety net for both mother and baby.

Preeclampsia is one of the leading complications of pregnancy worldwide, affecting up to 8 percent of all pregnancies.[59] The two most important diagnostic criteria for preeclampsia are an elevated blood pressure (hypertension) and excessive urinary protein excretion. If allowed to go untreated, preeclampsia can progress to *eclampsia,* which, while uncommon, is characterized by seizures and rarely, stroke.[60] Both preeclampsia and eclampsia are associated with an increased risk of poor pregnancy outcome, so preterm delivery is recommended when medical management has failed. This is true of other pregnancy complications as well, including intrauterine growth restriction, gestational diabetes, placenta previa, and other complications beyond the scope of this book.

Occasionally, the amniotic membranes surrounding the developing baby rupture prematurely. Whatever the cause, premature rupture of the may be appropriate. Pediatricians generally gauge a preterm infant's level of risk in terms of his/her *corrected gestational age*. Using this framework, an eight-week-old infant born at 32 weeks' gestational age is actually 40-week *corrected gestational age*, or a full-term equivalent newborn. Thus, preterm infants should avoid public exposures slightly longer than full-term infants. My wife and I avoided public venues, including church attendance, for at least six weeks after the birth of each of our children.

CHAPTER 2. GROWTH, NUTRITION, AND BREASTFEEDING

The milk supply of breastfeeding women is limited in the first day or two after birth, so milk intake too is minimal. Primitive reflexes, such as the suck and swallow and rooting reflexes, promote successful breastfeeding and are generally mature in the full-term infant, but these reflexes are less well developed in preterm infants. Full-term infants typically have adequate glucose stores (in the liver) to maintain normal blood sugar levels during fasting states (between meals), whereas preterm and small for gestational age infants are more likely to develop low blood sugar levels between meals. If blood sugar screening tests are below a safe threshold, or if weight loss is excessive, your pediatrician may recommend supplemental feedings with a commercial cow's milk formula—if only for a few days—until mother's transitional milk comes in.

The First Few Days

In the first day (or two) after birth, the breastfed newborn is content with as little as one teaspoon (5 milliliters) of colostrum per breastfeeding session. Soon, the healthy newborn arouses with signs of hunger (rooting, cueing) every two to three hours. Within two to five days, the transitional breastmilk begins to come in, the breasts become engorged, and the weight lost in those first few days is regained. Colostrum has a higher protein content, with milk that is typically bright yellow in color. As the transitional milk comes in, it changes to a pale-yellow color. Transitional milk is higher in fat and sugar and persists for as long as two weeks. Within 15 days, the mature milk, which is higher in lactose (sugar), comes in and has more of a creamy white color. The caloric density of breastmilk varies, ranging from 17 to 19 kcal/ounce.[29] Commercial cow's milk formulas, which were developed to mimic breastmilk, are fortified with vitamins and minerals, and with a few exceptions are enriched to 20 kcal/ounce. The use of preterm formulas, which are fortified to either 22 or 24 kcal/ounce, should be directed by a physician, as improper mixing can be harmful—always mix formula as directed by your physician or according to the instructions on the package insert/container.

Feeding Choice: Breastmilk vs. Commercial Formulas

Breastmilk is unquestionably superior to commercially available infant formulas—and we will discuss the benefits of breastfeeding later. However, personal circumstances may interfere with one's desire to breastfeed. If you are in this camp and are unable to breastfeed, your feeding choice should be respected and supported by the healthcare team. Despite the benefits of breastfeeding, formula-fed infants live long, meaningful, and productive lives—I am living proof! It is certainly appropriate for healthcare providers to encourage healthy choices, and breastfeeding is no exception, but each family has its own challenges and preferences, and your feeding choice should be honored for what it is—*your choice, for your baby, for your reasons*. Moreover, there are many ways to optimize your newborn's health and development, and some of these will be discussed in the chapters that follow. In the meantime, let us examine some of the fundamentals of newborn feeding, growth, and nutrition.

The healthy newborn feeds on demand, around the clock, for as long as 12 to 16 weeks—sometimes longer. Each newborn is different, but most develop a fairly consistent feeding pattern within the first week. During the first day (or so), your newborn may need to be aroused from sleep and stimulated for meals. Soon, however, the healthy newborn awakens hungry every two to three hours around the clock. Meals are typically followed by a period of *quiet contentment*, and thereafter by a period of sleep—only to repeat the cycle within two to three hours. This cycle varies from baby to baby, depending on the feeding choice and home environment, but breastfed newborns generally feed more frequently. Whereas breast-fed newborns feed as often as 10 to 12 times per day, formula-fed infants may feed only 8 to 10 times per day. Regardless of your feeding choice, interruptions to this cycle can have consequences, including irritability and feeding difficulties—so every effort should be made to minimize such interruptions. Breastfeeding attempts should be limited to 10 to 15 minutes at each breast, as most lactation specialists recommend limiting breastfeeding attempts to 30 minutes total. This minimizes the risk of sore, inflamed nipples, which can interfere with breastfeeding success.

Voiding and stooling patterns also vary from baby to baby and depend on a number of factors, including feeding choice and maternal diet. If intake is poor (i.e., from delayed lactation), then voiding and stooling will follow the same pattern. Regardless of feeding choice, newborns should have at least one void (wet diaper) within the first 24 hours and at least one stool (meconium counts) within the first 48 hours. Breastmilk stools are often described as yellow and seedy, while those of formula-fed infants are typically brown in color and pasty. If these basic "plumbing" milestones are not attained, then discharge should be delayed while the pediatrician performs a close examination of the genitalia and explores probable causes.

Oral Motor Development and Nutritional Intake

The ability to suck, swallow, and breathe, in coordinated fashion, is an intrinsic reflex—one that matures with each day that passes. However, not all infants of the same gestational age are the same. Some have more mature oral feeding skills than others. As noted previously, infants born preterm are more likely to develop low blood sugar levels (hypoglycemia). Therefore, preterm infants should have a screening blood sugar check

14

within two hours of birth. If the blood sugar level is low (< 40 mg/dL), then supplementation with glucose gel or formula may be needed until breastmilk intake improves or blood sugar levels have stabilized. The combination of low blood sugar levels and poor oral feeding skills requires vigilance by the healthcare team, especially among infants born preterm or small for gestational age.[30] Fortification (enrichment) of expressed breastmilk (or formula) to a higher caloric density (22 or 24 kcal/ounce) may be needed in extreme cases. For these reasons, monitoring intake, voiding and stooling patterns, and weight gain are appropriate in the first few days of life. Large for gestational age (LGA) newborns and infants born to diabetic mothers are more likely to require intravenous fluids (containing glucose) to maintain normal blood sugar levels.

Newborns can lose as much as 5 to 7 percent of their birth weight in the first three to five days—especially exclusively breastfed infants. Thus, your baby's medical team will determine whether nutritional intake is adequate based on daily weights, feeding, voiding and stooling patterns, and perhaps other indirect signs of adequate intake. Unfortunately, the volume of breastmilk ingested varies significantly between mother-baby pairs. The vast majority of newborns are 5 to 7 percent below their birth weight at hospital discharge. As such, the daily weight is one of the most objective measures of nutritional intake

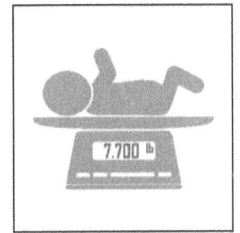
ID 127015201 ©Takt818 | Dreamstime.com

available to the medical team. As long as there is some evidence for adequate intake and weight loss is less than 8 to 10 percent of the birth weight, most pediatricians will permit discharge—with close outpatient follow-up. Breast engorgement suggests a significant increase in the transitional milk supply. Likewise, softening of the engorged breast after breastfeeding sessions, the presence of milk in the baby's mouth, and the audible sound of milk being swallowed are objective signs that breastmilk is being ingested. On the other hand, if weight loss exceeds 8 to 10 percent of the birth weight and one or more of these signs are absent, then supplementation with formula should be considered and discharge delayed.

Supplementation with formula. Supplementation is usually needed for less than two to three days, or until the transitional milk supply is sufficient to document an increase in weight gain. The frequency and volume of supplemental formula needed are determined by the degree of weight loss and the quality (or quantity) of bottle feedings. The daily weight trend and number of wet (or soiled) diapers provides a crude measure of intake. As a rule, the breast-fed newborn should continue to be placed at the breast with each feeding session - to stimulate milk production. Supplemental formula can be offered after removal from the breast based on the clinical circumstances (i.e., blood sugar level and/or degree of weight loss). The pediatrician and/or nursing staff will establish early feeding goals, but healthy newborns should be allowed to feed ad lib, on demand, around the clock. Supplementation with formula should be viewed as a *short-term solution to a short-term problem*. Given enough time and patience, the vast majority of newborns will breastfeed successfully. Consultative support from a certified lactation consultant (CLC) can be helpful in these circumstances.

> Supplementation with formula should be viewed as a short-term solution to a short-term problem, as the vast majority of infants go on to breastfeed successfully.

Infants born preterm or small for gestational age (SGA) may need additional calories for catch-up growth. Preterm breastmilk is deficient in nutrients that are important for bone mineralization, so your pediatrician may recommend replacing one or more breastmilk feedings with formula each day for two to four weeks. Alternatively, expressed breastmilk can be fortified with careful measurements of powdered formula. For example, two

However, each mother-baby pair is different, so if one position does not work, then try another, or reach out to a lactation specialist for support.

The key to breastfeeding success is consistently placing the baby at the breast every two to three hours until the transitional milk comes in. Each breastfeeding attempt stimulates milk production and ejection, so each attempt brings breastfeeding success that much closer. What may seem an unproductive breastfeeding session is actually a crucial step toward breastfeeding success. Stroking the breast and nipple stimulates hormone centers within the brain that promote milk production and ejection. Likewise, the sound of your newborn's cry stimulates milk production. In time, with repeated stimulation of lactation centers in the brain, the milk supply increases, the physiologic "let-down" occurs, and ever-increasing volumes of transitional milk are available. As the transitional milk comes in, the breasts become engorged—and evacuation of the breast provides relief. With each attempt, then, your newborn is more satisfied, and the cycle is completed. For some mother-infant pairs, the flow of milk can be so fast as to overwhelm the newborn's still immature suck and swallow reflexes, so caution is recommended at the beginning of feeding attempts. Once again, consistently putting the baby to breast is the most effective way to achieve breastfeeding success.

Challenges that accompany breastfeeding. While the benefits of breastfeeding are numerous, so too are the challenges! One of the most challenging aspects of breastfeeding is determining the volume of milk ingested with early breastfeeding sessions. Infants who fail to awaken spontaneously should be aroused, stimulated, and put to breast (or offered formula), as newborns are often sleepy in the first hours after birth. As discussed in the previous section, skin-to-skin care has been shown to promote both mother-infant bonding and breastfeeding success—so it is important to capitalize on this concept.[32] Unfortunately, delayed milk production is common after cesarean section (and other pregnancy complications), so vigilance may be needed to ensure the newborn receives adequate nourishment. Nursing mothers should drink plenty of water and rest as much as possible between breastfeeding sessions. While breast shields can provide relief from mild discomfort, a commercial-grade breast pump can provide relief when the nipples/areola become sore or inflamed or when the lactiferous ducts become infected (mastitis). Painful breastfeeding attempts should prompt a call to your obstetrician for evaluation. If you are diagnosed with mastitis, a bacterial infection of the lactiferous ducts, it is appropriate to "pump and dump" the breastmilk for a few days while undergoing treatment with antibiotics.

Postpartum fatigue. Aside from the difficulties that accompany delayed milk production and ensuring adequate intake, maternal fatigue is quite common.[41] In one study, postpartum fatigue was significant among first-pregnancy breastfeeding women.[42] Overall, the medical literature does not support a clear correlation between feeding choice (breast vs. formula) and maternal fatigue. However, maternal fatigue is frequently reported among nursing mothers.[41] Given the demands of breastfeeding on demand, every two to three hours around the clock, for as long as 12 to 16 weeks, it is no surprise that postpartum fatigue is so common! Unfortunately, postpartum fatigue increases the risk of co-bedding and therefore the risk of sleep-related infant death.

Postpartum fatigue, co-bedding, and sleep-related deaths. Co-bedding (sleeping in the same bed with your baby) is a significant temptation when fatigue sets in. The human body needs roughly 6 hours of sleep in a 24-hour period. However, breastfeeding does not leave much time for sleep. If not for the joys of motherhood, most women would collapse from exhaustion! Unfortunately, the risk of sudden unexpected infant death (SUID) increases substantially with co-bedding, and several sleep-related

22

risk factors have been documented in the medical literature. For now, consider that postpartum fatigue presents a significant challenge, and preparing for this challenge is an important aspect of caring for your newborn. Develop a contingency plan when you sense fatigue setting in. Ask your spouse or partner for help, or if you are a single mother, and have no one to turn to, then simply lay the baby down (in the supine position). If necessary, let the baby fuss while you take a nap. But whatever you do, DO NOT fall asleep with the baby!

Reasons to avoid breastfeeding. Finally, there are several important medical reasons to avoid breastfeeding. If you have been diagnosed with tuberculosis (TB), human immunodeficiency virus (HIV), or leprosy, you should abstain from breastfeeding.[43] While rare, these infections are associated with an increased risk of transmission to the newborn. On the other hand, *hepatitis A, B, and C are all generally safe for breastfeeding*, unless the nipples are cracked or bleeding or open lesions are observed on the breast, nipple, or areola.[43] Infants born to hepatitis B-infected women should receive hepatitis B immune globulin (HBIG) and the first of three doses of the hepatitis B vaccine series before initiating breastfeeding. If the nipples become cracked or there are open/bleeding lesions on the breast, refrain from breastfeeding until the lesions have healed, which generally takes 10–14 days, and there is no risk of ingesting maternal blood from the breast. Likewise, breastfeeding should be avoided in the context of a diagnosis of mastitis, an infection of the lactiferous ducts within the breast.

CHAPTER 3. SLEEP, HUMAN INTERACTION, AND BRAIN DEVELOPMENT

Despite advances in medical science, we still have much to learn about the effects of environmental stress on the developing brain. There is, however, some evidence that both sleep and the social environment contribute to healthy brain development. The newborn brain is structurally and functionally immature at birth, even among healthy, full-term newborns. Brain growth peaks in the first three to six months of life.[44] Moreover, early life exposures, including sleep, mother-baby interactions, and environmental exposures, have been shown to have a significant impact on brain function and development.

Synaptogenesis, a term used by researchers to signify the formation of connections within the brain, peaks at about four months of age and continues until the third year of life or perhaps longer.[45] This means that connections linked with human development peak during the newborn period. Likewise, sensory information in the first weeks and months of life stimulates the fine-tuning and electrical circuitry of the brain—a process known as *patterning*. Synaptogenesis and patterning are highly active in the first weeks and months after birth, and both prenatal and postnatal events are believed to impact these important developmental processes.[45] The take-home point is that early life experiences, both positive and negative, appear to impact newborn brain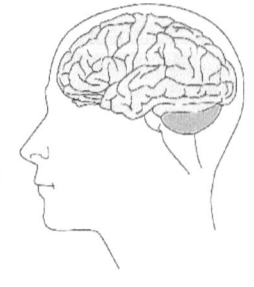

by OpenClipart-Vectors via Pixabay

development. One of the ways you can positively impact your newborn's development is to provide a healthy routine and a nurturing home environment.

Establishing a routine

Newborns are surprisingly consistent in their feeding patterns, often establishing a routine within the first week of life. Learning to recognize the signals (cues) that your baby is hungry, sleepy, or in need of a diaper change is essential to establishing a routine. Minor modifications are unavoidable, and there is no need to fret about minor interruptions to the cycle. On the other hand, newborns thrive on healthy routines. So, household activities should be planned around the newborn's schedule and mother's need for rest. Since feeding and soiling patterns often coincide, even diaper changes can be scheduled to a degree. Changing the baby's diaper as soon as 30 to 45 minutes after a meal, but before the next sleep cycle, will ensure that your baby goes down for a nap clean and dry. There is a natural rhythm to feeding, bonding, and stooling, and embracing this rhythm can facilitate healthy sleep/wake cycles and brain development. In time, this rhythm becomes so organic that interruptions can affect a newborn's sense of well-being. An old adage seems appropriate here: "Never wake a sleeping baby!"

Sleep and newborn development. Sleep is essential for normal brain function and development. Newborns awaken hungry every two to three hours, followed by a period of quiet contentment, and soon thereafter by a period of sleep lasting as long as one to three hours. Most newborns sleep between 16 and 18 hours per day in the first days and weeks after birth, some longer. During this time, the developing brain is actively forming new connections and pruning existing ones.[46, 47] Each newborn is different, of course, and the home environment can affect this cycle in both positive and negative ways. Anything that interferes with this rhythm can have adverse effects on your newborn. The manifestations of stress are often subtle but include yawning, rapid or shallow breathing, mottling of the skin, tremors, arching, and hiccupping. Importantly, the absence of sleep can lead to irritability, the ultimate manifestation of stress in a newborn. One or more of these signs of stress suggests the possibility that either your newborn has had inadequate sleep or the environment is unsuitable for sleep and healthy brain development.

> Sleep is essential for normal brain function and development. During sleep, the brain is actively forming new connections and pruning existing ones.

Newborns generally sleep through the night by the fourth month after birth. Some are still feeding around the clock for as long as four to six months, so this is an extremely challenging period. Establishing a routine is one of the most important ways you can encourage your newborn to sleep through the night. A supportive partner can play a huge role. By keeping diaper stations fully stocked and/or delivering a hungry baby to an often-fatigued mother, the supportive partner is contributing to the health and well-being of both mother and baby. Likewise, assisting with diaper changes, burping the baby after meals, and returning the baby to the portable bassinette after meals are practical ways your partner can provide support. Even the most devoted mother can fall asleep while feeding a baby at 3:00 a.m., which increases the risk of accidental suffocation. Therefore, I recommend establishing a positive, supportive accountability system to ensure that your newborn is returned to the bassinette before you fall asleep. One of my deepest regrets as a husband and father is not being more supportive during these long, difficult nights. If you are so unfortunate as to have a knucklehead partner like me, consider setting your phone to alarm 15 to 20 minutes after the start of each feeding session—but avoid co-bedding with the baby!

> Establishing a routine is one of the most important ways you can encourage your newborn to sleep through the night.

symptomatic despite the usual measures. Most infants recover by their first birthday, and the vast majority of the rest recover by age three years.[128, 133] Lactose intolerance is an intolerance to the sugar component of milk, which is extremely rare in the newborn period and usually develops after the second year of life.

Colic. The term *colic* describes periods of intense irritability and crying in the newborn period. Among the most challenging conditions encountered in infancy, colic affects as many as 40 percent of all newborns, peaking at around six weeks of age.[138] Colic is often *defined* by the "rule of three": crying or irritability for more than *three hours* per day, for more than *three days* per week, and for at least *three weeks*.[139] The first and most important thing to remember is that colic is a benign, self-limited condition. In other words, colic is a short-lived problem that eventually passes without consequence. Episodes occur at roughly the same time of day and with the same intensity. However, infants with colic continue to have all the usual signs of well-being, with one exception—irritability. Episodes of colic may be accompanied by "gas" and other nonspecific gastrointestinal signs, but this may not be the *cause* of irritability. Some feel that gassy spells are the result of excessive swallowing of air, not the cause of the condition.

> Colic is a diagnosis of exclusion, meaning that other important causes of irritability (inconsolable crying) should be ruled out before considering the diagnosis of colic.

The majority of infants with colic have extended periods of normalcy, without crying or irritability, and have many of the usual signs of well-being, including a good appetite, periods of quiet contentment, and normal sleep and behavior. While colic is a benign, self-limited condition, the acute onset of inconsolable crying is concerning and should prompt an evaluation for causes of pain, including infectious disorders. A brief list of potential causes of pain or irritability should be considered, including gastroesophageal reflux disease (GERD), infections of the bones or joints, meningitis, intestinal obstruction, testicular torsion, hair-tourniquet syndrome, corneal abrasion, and even long-bone fracture. The initial evaluation is important, and for this reason pediatricians generally consider colic a *diagnosis of exclusion*, meaning that the diagnosis is generally not established until other, more concerning causes of inconsolable crying have been ruled out.[139]

The difficulty, of course, is differentiating colic from other, more serious causes of pain or irritability. It is generally not necessary to perform elaborate or expensive diagnostic investigations, especially if other signs of well-being are present. We have already established that appetite is the most important sign of well-being. Does your baby still have a good appetite and adequate intake? Other signs of well-being may include periods of quiet contentment after a meal and relatively normal sleep/wake cycles. The otherwise healthy newborn should have other signs of well-being, and colic is no exception to this rule. Because the acute onset of irritability has serious implications, the initial steps of the diagnostic workup are best performed by an experienced pediatrician, one capable of making a diagnosis without ordering an infinite number of diagnostic tests. For the experienced pediatrician, this evaluation is fairly routine.

Once the diagnosis of colic has been established, a systematic elimination of potential triggers should begin. If you are breastfeeding, consider eliminating dairy products, chocolate, certain fruits, and vegetables—one at a time. Do not, however, discontinue a medication without first consulting your physician. Another potential cause of colic is *overstimulation*, including television and radio, or loud noises unique to your home and family. Irritability may simply be a sign that your baby needs more rest and/or less chaos. Most parents are able to identify triggers, as well as certain positions or activities (e.g., rocking motions) that "settle" the colicky baby. There is some evidence favoring the use of probiotics in the management of colic, but the evidence is not conclusive. Some studies favor the use of probiotics, while others do not.[138] Unfortunately, there is no "magic bullet" for treating colic. Warm blankets, gentle rocking motions, soft music, and a quiet room have all been used successfully, but your baby may have unique needs. While a good pediatrician is a valued partner, you are uniquely qualified to identify the most important triggers!

The challenge for many parents is accepting the reassurance that colic will pass. The most important concept, and perhaps the most difficult, is the exercise of *patience*, as colic generally resolves within three months.[139] Caring for the colicky baby can be extremely stressful and may be more difficult for some than for others. If you find yourself caring for a baby with colic, develop enough self-awareness to ask for help when you are becoming stressed-out. Even the best parents can find themselves frustrated with prolonged crying spells. When you are frustrated or overwhelmed, the best policy is to simply lay the baby down and walk away to gather your nerves.[140] Reach out to a supportive friend or family member for help while you catch your breath. And remember, colic is a short-lived condition that passes with time. There is life after colic—and it will come sooner than you think.

Discolored stool. Generally speaking, the color of a newborn's stool is unimportant. However, there are a few exceptions, and these exceptions are generally accompanied by other signs or symptoms of illness. Whereas most breastfed newborns have yellow, seedy stools, formula-fed babies typically have stools that are more formed and vary from brown to green to dark tan in color. The color of a baby's stool, however, has more to do with the intestinal *microbiome* than anything else. The intestinal microbiome is an ever-evolving ecosystem of microorganisms that derives initially from the mother, including bacteria from the vaginal canal, maternal skin, breastfeeding, and microbial transfer that occurs during gestation.[141] This is a normal part of human physiology that is influenced by multiple environmental factors.[141] While our understanding of the human microbiome is growing, its impacts on human health and disease are still poorly understood. The point is that the color of a newborn's stool is related, in large part, to the newborn's intestinal microbiome, which is still poorly understood—so don't read too much into it!

Bright red (blood-streaked) stool. The two clear exceptions to this general rule are (1) bright red blood coming from the rectum, and (2) black, tarry stools—both of which are manifestations of intestinal bleeding. These conditions are discussed at length in appendix A, as both reflect the presence of intestinal bleeding that deserves a formal evaluation by a pediatric physician. That said, blood-tinged stools (i.e., blood streaks at the margin of the stool) in an otherwise well-appearing newborn generally suggest a benign or uncomplicated condition. Occasionally, but certainly less frequently, blood-streaked stools are the result of milk protein sensitivity, which was discussed in a previous section. Nonetheless, the presence of blood-streaked stools warrants a formal evaluation by a pediatrician, if only to *ensure* that the cause of bleeding is benign and uncomplicated. Newborns who have a good appetite, normal activity and sleep, normal growth, and are otherwise well-appearing usually have a benign, self-limited condition or one that can be addressed in the outpatient clinical setting.

The most common cause of blood-streaked stool is an anal fissure, a small tear or abrasion at the rectum. The rectal mucosa is thin, friable, and easily abraded by the passage of hard stool, excessive wiping, or even frequent stooling. This is true for older children and adults as well, but it is important to remember that rectal fissures may not be visible on examination of the diaper region. Anal fissures can be either external (visible on exam) or internal (not visible on exam). Importantly, internal fissures are no more serious than external fissures, but because they are not externally visible, they create something of a diagnostic dilemma. Other diagnostic studies may be needed to rule out other causes of blood in the stool, especially if large amounts of blood are noted. However, blood-tinged stools are often uncomplicated (benign) in the otherwise well-appearing newborn. The presence of bright red blood in the stool, especially in large quantities, warrants a thorough evaluation by a physician. Remember, also, that infants who fail to receive vitamin K before discharge have an increased risk of bleeding in the early postnatal period.

The maternal and perinatal history can aid in the diagnosis of blood-streaked stools, especially in the early postnatal period. Bloody stools within the first 24 hours suggest the possibility of swallowed maternal blood, which can result from one of several pregnancy-related conditions. Separation of the placenta from the uterine wall during active labor (placental abruption) is among the more common causes of swallowed maternal blood. Fortunately, tests for the presence of adult hemoglobin are available if needed.[142] However, the most important elements of the history are no different from what we have already discussed. Does your baby have all the usual signs of well-being? A vigorous appetite, normal activity and behavior, periods of quiet contentment after meals? A grossly bloody stool (blood mixed throughout the stool) warrants an immediate evaluation by a pediatrician, but a blood-streaked stool (small amounts of blood at the periphery of the stool) is less urgent and can generally be managed in the outpatient clinic.

Common Abnormalities of the Eyes and Ears

Clogged tear duct (nasolacrimal duct stenosis). Nasolacrimal duct stenosis is a benign condition characterized by a clear to cloudy mucoid drainage from the eyelids, which results from a narrowing (stenosis) or plugging of the nasolacrimal ducts with debris. The nasolacrimal duct is a narrow duct that connects the inner (medial) margins of the lower eyelids to the nasal sinuses. The presence of this duct is the reason we all have the sniffles (a runny nose) when crying or tearful. The most effective treatment is application of a warm compress and gentle massage, or pressure directed from the medial (midline) corner of the eye, down along the side of the nose. This gentle pressure "pushes" secretions through the nasolacrimal duct, thus encouraging the flow of drainage into the sinuses. If secretions become yellow or green, treatment with antimicrobial eye drops, like trimethoprim/polymyxin B or gentamicin ophthalmic, is appropriate. Otherwise, gentle massage with a warm compress along the medial aspect of the nose is generally effective.

Lazy eye (strabismus). Lazy eye is also common in the newborn period, and while generally benign, it should be followed carefully for the first several weeks to months after birth. Risk factors for lazy eye include prematurity and maternal smoking during pregnancy, but genetic predisposition may also play a role.[143-145] Sometimes called *strabismus* by pediatricians, lazy eye that persists beyond the four-month well-baby visit warrants referral to a pediatric ophthalmologist. Referral is important because persistence can lead to amblyopia, which can adversely impact visual acuity in the nondominant eye. That said, lazy eye is easily treated by an experienced pediatric ophthalmologist, and long-term outcomes are excellent.

Disconjugate gaze. Another condition that provokes parental anxiety in the first few weeks is sometimes referred to as *disconjugate gaze*, a condition in which one eye tracks objects appropriately while the other neglects the object tracked. Disconjugate gaze is most noticeable in the first few weeks but generally resolves within two to three months as the external muscles of the eye mature and gain strength. Both eyes should be tracking objects symmetrically (conjugately) within two months of birth, so failure of the eyes to track objects conjugately by four months of age warrants referral to a pediatric ophthalmologist. That said, the vast majority of infants track objects normally by four months of age.

PART II – A DEEPER DIVE INTO NEWBORN CARE

CHAPTER 8. INFANTS BORN EITHER PREMATURE OR SMALL FOR GESTATIONAL AGE

The majority of live births in developed countries are uncomplicated. Most infants are born full-term (39 to 40 weeks' gestation) with a normal birth weight (between 2,500 and 4,000 gm) and have an uncomplicated transition to postnatal life. That is, most newborns have a normal breathing pattern, normal posture and tone, and are pink within the first few minutes after birth. On occasion, minor complications are noted, including mild or transient respiratory distress, birth depression, or birth trauma. The vast majority, however, respond to gentle stimulation, suctioning of the mouth for secretions, and/or supplemental "blow-by" oxygen. Rarely, specialized care is needed to complete the initial transition to postnatal life, and this is especially true of infants born prematurely. Unfortunately, prematurity is largely unavoidable, resulting from either preterm labor or complications of pregnancy.

One out of every 10 to 12 live-born infants are born prematurely.[146] The vast majority of these are born between 34 and 37 weeks' gestation, otherwise known as the "late preterm" period.[1] Since most of the complications of prematurity are experienced by infants born less than 28 weeks' gestation, the vast majority of infants born preterm have favorable short- and long-term outcomes.[1, 146, 147]

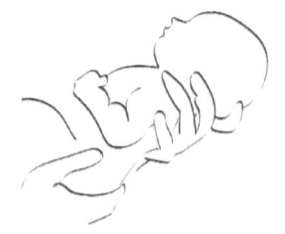

By ViancaVanDijk via Pixabay

However, not all infants of the same gestational age have the same outcomes. For example, survival and healthy brain development have improved substantially in recent years, even among those born at extreme gestations.[148, 149] Overall, however, infants born preterm are slightly more likely to have school difficulties, behavioral/social problems, and/or medical disabilities at school age—the lower the gestational age at birth, the greater the risk of adversity later in childhood.[150]

Late preterm (near-term) infants. While late preterm infants are born "just a few weeks early," they are still more likely than full-term infants to develop respiratory distress, temperature instability, low blood sugar, jaundice, or feeding problems.[1, 151] Mothers of late preterm infants are also more likely to have breastfeeding difficulties, including early breastfeeding cessation, than mothers who deliver full-term newborns.[13] To obtain adequate nutrition, the newborn must suck, swallow, and breathe in coordinated fashion without aspirating milk into the airway. Feeding is a complex developmental process that begins to emerge at around 33 to 34 weeks' gestation, sometimes later. Thus, depending on the gestational age at birth and circumstances of the pregnancy, some preterm infants are incapable of obtaining adequate nutrition without assistance. In these cases, either tube feedings (via nasogastric tube) or intravenous fluids may be needed, if only for a few days.

If tube feedings are needed, admission to the NICU is appropriate. The NICU nurse typically initiates small-volume feeds through a polyurethane or silicone nasogastric tube that is passed through the nose and down into the stomach. This allows the clinical team to provide *enteral* nutrition while awaiting oral feeding skills to develop, which may also mitigate the need for intravenous fluids. Depending on the gestational age, maturation of primitive reflexes (suck, swallow, and breathe) can take days to weeks to develop. Like so many other developmental processes, a tincture of time is all that is needed. Most infants are taking full-volume oral feeds by 36 to 37 weeks' gestational age—three to four weeks before the baby's due date!

Immature suck and swallow correlate with other signs of developmental immaturity as well, including transient drops in heart rate and/or oxygen saturation. Sometimes referred to as *bradycardia* or *desaturation spells*, these cardiopulmonary events are evidence of physiologic immaturity. While these "spells" are common in preterm infants, they also suggest a slight increase in the risk of a life-threatening event, and for this reason, most pediatricians and neonatologists require that infants demonstrate at least three but as many as five spell-free days before discharge is deemed safe. This is often frustrating for parents, as the slightly small, slightly preterm newborn may appear normal in every other way, including the coordination of suck and swallow, the ability to take full-volume feeds, and the ability to maintain a normal core body temperature in an open crib. Nonetheless, this period of observation is an important means of ensuring the baby has achieved sufficient physiologic stability for a safe discharge.[1]

On occasion, infants are born smaller than their peers born at the same gestational age. These small for gestational age (SGA) infants share some of the same difficulties as preterm infants. For example, infants born to women with high blood pressure or preeclampsia may have intrauterine growth restriction (IUGR), which results in less subcutaneous body mass. Subcutaneous body mass is important for maintaining a normal core body temperature. Temperature instability is common, so a radiant heat source (a crib with an external radiant heat source) or an isolette (incubator) may be needed to maintain normal body temperature. As discussed earlier, small for gestational age newborns also have limited glycogen stores, which are important for maintaining normal blood sugar levels in fasting states (between meals). Likewise, infants with low blood sugar may require intravenous fluids (with glucose) or supplemental formula feedings to maintain normal blood sugar levels. Generally speaking, infants born at less than 35 weeks' gestation and those born less than 2,000 grams (4 lb. 6.4 oz.) require admission to the NICU.

> Mothers of late preterm infants are at greater risk for breastfeeding difficulties, including early breastfeeding cessation.

The Neonatal Resuscitation Program (NRP) was established to guide physicians and practitioners in the care of newborns during the critical transition from fetal to newborn life. Most hospitals have protocols incorporating NRP guidelines into their delivery room practices. For premature newborns, these guidelines focus largely on temperature regulation, thresholds for advanced respiratory support, and the administration of intravenous fluids and medications. Given the challenges of preterm birth, a great deal of research has been conducted to improve the care and outcomes of high-risk newborns. One of the most important lessons from the past two decades of research is that preterm infants tend to have better outcomes when born in centers that standardize as many elements as possible, especially care in the delivery room and early postnatal period.[152]

Unfortunately, the effectiveness of medical care varies widely in neonatal intensive care units, and large differences in outcomes have been noted among birthing centers.[153-155] Research suggests that differences in the outcomes most important to parents (survival and development) may be related to differences in the quality of care. There is evidence, for example, that high-volume centers (centers caring for more than 50 preterm infants per year) have better outcomes than low-volume centers.[89] Ideally, infants born less than 32 weeks' gestation and those with anticipated medical or surgical complications should be delivered in birthing centers that employ nurses and physicians experienced in the care of high-risk newborns. Unfortunately, some things are out of your control, including the onset of labor. So, while it is ideal to deliver a high-risk babies in a high-volume centers, it is also better to deliver in a low-volume center than in the back of an automobile or ambulance! Thus, if you have a high-risk pregnancy or anticipate delivering a high-risk newborn, consider developing a plan for delivery and/or transfer to a qualified birthing center.

Most states in the US restrict the care of infants born at less than 32 weeks' gestation to hospitals capable of providing such care. Level I perinatal centers are generally limited to the care of healthy newborns who are at least 35 weeks' gestation (late preterm infants) and those who require only minimal care beyond that of a healthy newborn. Level II nurseries, on the other hand, are permitted to provide care for moderately ill newborns, including the temporary provision of advanced respiratory support, with guidance and support from level III and IV neonatal intensive care units in the region. If you have questions about the capabilities of the hospital nearest you, it is reasonable to ask your obstetrician about the most appropriate hospital for delivery.

CHAPTER 9. SUDDEN UNEXPECTED INFANT DEATH

I include this chapter on a somewhat frightening topic in the hope that I can help at least one family avoid a terrifying, life-altering outcome. My aim, then, is to minimize the risk of a *potentially avoidable* adverse outcome, not to frighten you. If, on the other hand, this topic elicits anxiety, consider skipping this chapter and instead search the internet for "safe sleep" recommendations provided by the American Academy of Pediatrics—these recommendations have been credited with decreasing the rate of sudden unexpected death in the US.[11] To provide context for these recommendations, allow me to share a brief review of the history of infant mortality in the US.

Infant death rates are relatively low in contemporary US history, but this has not always been so. In colonial America, as many as 30 percent of infants died before their first birthday, and most families experienced the loss of at least one child in the first year.[156] Fortunately, infant mortality began to decline in the late nineteenth century; and by the late twentieth century the likelihood of infant death had dropped from roughly one out of every 10 live births to one out of every 100.[157] Currently, less than one out of every 1,000 infants die each year, most in the first month of life.[158] Improvements in survival have been attributed to a cleaner milk supply and to other public policy efforts, including hand hygiene and childhood vaccines.[159, 160] Although maternal and newborn health have improved substantially since the early twentieth century, the majority of infant deaths still occur within the *neonatal period*—the first 28 days after birth.[54, 158]

Each year, approximately 3,600 infants die unexpectedly from sleep-related deaths in the US.[11] Since the late 1960s, the term *sudden infant death syndrome* (SIDS) has been used to describe the sudden death of a child less than one year of age—that remains unexplained after a thorough investigation. In recent years, sleep-related deaths have been categorized more broadly as *sudden unexpected infant death* (SUID), which includes SIDS *plus* accidental suffocation and other unknown causes.[161] In 2022, there were 3700 deaths from SUID, 1529 from SIDS, 1040 from accidental suffocation (co-bedding), and 1131 from unknown causes.[162] While the annual rate of SUID has decreased significantly since the AAP released information on safe sleep practices, it still remains one of the leading causes of infant death in the western world.[163, 164]

Despite advances in research, unknown causes of infant death continue to plague pediatricians and public health officials. Fortunately, researchers have identified several important risk factors, and this chapter was added to disseminate knowledge in the hope of decreasing the risk of SUID further. The risk of SUID is significantly greater among preterm infants than among infants born full-term and decreases incrementally with increasing gestational age.[165-167] In 1994 a group of researchers proposed that the brainstem may be more vulnerable in some newborns than others. According to this theory, a newborn's underlying vulnerability peaks at a critical stage of development, but increases with factors such as sleep position, secondhand smoke, prematurity, environmental temperature, or perhaps even the "common cold".[168] While this is plausible, many questions remain, and the National Institutes of Health (NIH) continues to fund research into this complex public health issue.

Brief Resolved Unexplained Events (BRUE). Formerly known as apparent life-threatening events (ALTE), the AAP has proposed a change in terminology regarding apparent life-threatening events (ALTE). Using the former definition, an ALTE was "frightening to the observer and characterized by the cessation of breathing (apnea), a change in skin color, abnormal muscle tone, and either choking or gagging. Using the new and improved definition, a BRUE is an event that is *brief*, i.e., less than 1 minute, resolved at the time of presentation, and unexplained.[169] Using this definition, the AAPs clinical practice guideline states that a BRUE is characterized by (1) cyanosis (a blue discoloration of the skin) or pallor, (2) absent, decreased, or irregular breathing, 3) a marked change in tone (either hyper- or hypotonia), and (4) an altered level of consciousness.[169]

By definition, then, ALTEs and BRUEs do not result in death of a child but suggest the possibility of an increased risk of a future life-threatening event. BRUE are further characterized as either low risk or high risk, based on risk factors identified in the history and physical examination. Infants categorized as high-risk BRUE warrant further investigation; low-risk infants do not. In the development of the most recent practice guideline, the AAP identified the following risk factors that place infants in the high-risk category: 1) infants less than 2 months of age, 2) those with a history of prematurity, 3) and those with a history of more than one event.[169] Additionally, infants born less than 32 weeks' gestation and those who require cardiopulmonary resuscitation are deemed at greater risk.[169]

The evidence upon which these recommendations are based derives from numerous studies and countless hours of AAP committee work. The following is merely a brief summary of the available evidence, which appears to be growing each year. In a large population-based study of infants born in Austria, roughly 2.5 infants per 1,000 live births presented to the emergency room after an apparent life-threatening event (ALTE).[170] Preterm infants are two to three times more likely to die of SUID than infants born full-term, so parents of preterm infants should exercise extreme vigilance with regard to safe sleep.[165] While infants born less than 29 weeks' gestation (or less than 1,500 gm) are at greatest risk, late preterm infants (34 to 37 weeks) are at greater risk than infants born full-term.[166] However, a number of other factors contribute to the risk of BRUE (formerly

ALTE) and SUID, and some are *potentially avoidable*—*yet* another reason for including this chapter in an otherwise optimistic book on newborn care!

Temperature regulation and SUID. As much as 85 percent of heat loss in newborns occurs at the head and scalp, so knitted caps have long been used to minimize heat loss, especially in the first few days after birth. However, there is now some evidence that elevated environmental temperatures and heat stress may increase the risk of SUID/SIDS.[171] In one study, infants who were heavily wrapped and those left in rooms in which the heat was left on overnight were more likely to die of SIDS.[171] The study found no association between viral infections *alone* and SIDS, but those with the combination of a viral infection and over-bundling were at greater risk.[171] While these studies are inconclusive, over-bundling and sleep in poorly ventilated rooms have been associated with an increased risk of SUID, and exposure to a viral infection *may* increase this risk. It seems prudent, then, to avoid extreme environmental temperatures, over-bundling, and poorly ventilated rooms when laying your newborn down to sleep. Moreover, infants with signs of a viral upper respiratory infection, or cold, should be monitored carefully during periods of sleep.

Sleep position and SUID. While the evidence for the above recommendations is weak, the evidence regarding proper positioning during sleep (i.e., on the back) is quite strong. In a study of infants that died of SIDS in Chicago, the following factors were associated with SUID/SIDS: *prone* sleep position, soft sleeping surfaces, use of pillows, bed sharing, and failure to use a pacifier.[172] In 2016 the American Academy of Pediatrics provided an update supporting safe sleep practices.[11] This comprehensive summary included evidence that prone (face down) and side-lying sleep positions appear to increase the risk of re-breathing expired carbon dioxide, which in turn results in carbon dioxide retention and low oxygen levels. Prone and side-lying positioning also appear to increase the risk of overheating and alter the body's control of the cardiovascular system during sleep.[11, 172] The *Back to Sleep* program, advocated by both the American Academy of Pediatrics and the American College of Pediatricians, resulted from these and other research findings.[11, 173]

> Safe sleep summarized: avoid prone and side-lying positions, avoid soft bedding and materials, avoid co-bedding (sleeping in the same bed), and avoid overheating and over-bundling.

Most newborn deaths related to accidental suffocation occur within the first four months of life.[165] Accidental suffocation can happen to anyone. Maternal fatigue has been implicated as a risk factor, especially in the first few weeks after birth, and maternal fatigue affects parents of every race, ethnicity, and social class. "Safe sleep" refers to the following sleep practices: avoiding prone and side-lying positions, avoiding soft bedding and materials, avoiding co-bedding (sleeping in the same bed), and avoiding overheating and over-bundling.[11] Consider, also, the importance of managing postpartum fatigue and ensuring an optimal sleep environment. The available evidence suggests that safe sleep also includes avoiding extreme temperatures and ensuring that your newborn sleeps in a well-ventilated room, free of secondhand smoke.[11] Develop a safety plan before leaving the hospital, and ask for help *when* fatigue sets in. These are some very practical ways that you can support the health and well-being of your newborn.

Home apnea monitoring. Unfortunately, research has failed to show any tangible benefits to home apnea monitoring.[174] While preterm infants have a slightly greater risk of SUID than those born full-term, apnea of prematurity, which is common among infants born less than 34 weeks' gestation, is not a reliable predictor of SUID. Home apnea monitors are appropriate for technology-dependent infants and infants with complex medical conditions—especially those requiring home oxygen. Good pediatricians promote *proven* safe sleep practices, such as "back to sleep", use of firm sleeping surfaces, and avoidance of co-bedding and secondhand smoke. Finally, please implement safe sleep practices immediately after delivery, and have open conversations with friends and family members who may be assisting in the care of your newborn. In so doing, you will decrease the risk of a potentially avoidable adverse outcome!

CHAPTER 10. INFANTS WITH DISABILITIES

Given the wide range of moral and religious values, it is not surprising that there is a wide range of opinions regarding the care of infants with disabilities. However, I make no apologies for my view that each child is made in the image of God, deserving the same rights and protections as you and me, regardless of his/her mental or physical capacity. In the paragraphs that follow, I will demonstrate, with support from epidemiologic research, that children and adults with disabilities have a more favorable view of their own quality of life than suggested by existing medical dogma, including children born preterm.[175]

Although less than 5 percent of infants are born with birth defects or disabilities, as many as 15 percent of children (ages three to seventeen) have one or more disabilities.[3] Disabilities are so common, in fact, that you probably know someone who either has or cares for a child or adult with a physical or developmental disability.[3, 176] Unfortunately, I have witnessed the emotional distress of families facing this reality, and these conversations have been among the most difficult of my career.

Learning disabilities, attention deficit and hyperactivity disorder (ADHD), and autism represent the vast majority of disabilities in childhood—many of them *minor* disabilities that go unrecognized by the casual observer. Data from a population-based study, published in 2015, suggests that the prevalence of cerebral palsy, intellectual disability, hearing loss, and visual impairment have remained relatively stable over time, whereas that of autistic spectrum disorder appears to be increasing.[177] In a large study of children with disabilities, subjects were classified into three groups—those with autism spectrum disorder *with* intellectual disability, those with autism spectrum disorder *without* intellectual disability, and those with intellectual disability *without* autism spectrum disorder. Children in all three groups had higher rates of preterm birth, low birth weight, or low Apgar score.[178] Unfortunately, prematurity and low Apgar score are largely unavoidable.[179, 180] The good news, however, is that most preterm infants are born after 32 weeks' gestation and have either mild or no disabilities at all.[181] And while low APGAR score is sometimes associated with a greater risk of intellectual disability, it is also less common than prematurity.[182]

Whatever the cause, learning that a child may have a physical or intellectual disability can be traumatic. Although the vast majority of disabilities are minor, some are severe and occasionally life-altering. That said, I bring a more optimistic view than many healthcare professionals, and my optimism is supported by clinical experience and by evidence from the pediatric literature. Despite the challenges that accompany physical or intellectual disabilities, many children (and their families) have an overall *favorable* quality of life. And while it is true that the medical literature provides some conflicting evidence, there appears to be a growing body of evidence that supports my view.

In a study published in 2014, parents reported significantly higher health-related quality of life among children with disabilities than was predicted by physicians on formal screening tests.[183] While physicians anticipated medical complications and focused on the burdens to caregivers, parents expressed optimism overall.[183] In the same year, researchers conducted a systematic review of the medical literature, examining over 400 quality of life publications.[184] Regardless of the disability or testing instrument chosen, the majority of children reported quality of life ratings *similar* to those in the general population.[184] The one exception was that children with disabilities often reported lower scores in the physical functioning/health domain. Another study included roughly 500 children with cerebral palsy in Europe. Children with cerebral palsy had self-reported quality of life that was similar to that of children in the general population in all functional domains except *schooling*.[185] In yet another study, self-reported health status and quality of life among children with cerebral palsy in Ontario was described as "excellent" or "very good" by 57 percent of youth and 46 percent of adults.[186]

Therefore, if healthcare professionals' views regarding infants with disabilities are based on a perception that children with special needs have poor quality of life, then these perceptions are flawed. Quality of life ratings for children with disabilities are often *similar* to those of children without developmental disabilities.[184, 186] Consider trisomy 21 (Down syndrome), the most common chromosomal abnormality in live-born infants.[187] Children with trisomy 21 have an extra copy of chromosome 21 and are frequently born with one or more end-organ abnormalities, including congenital heart disease, glaucoma (high pressure within the eye), thyroid disorders, intestinal anomalies, and developmental delay. Although children with Down syndrome have lower *health-related* quality of life than children without Down syndrome, the large majority of adults with Down syndrome have favorable self-reported quality of life ratings.[188] The good news, then, is that children with physical and developmental disabilities can and frequently do live long, meaningful, and productive lives.

The prevailing bias against children with disabilities. Despite a growing body of evidence that children and adults with disabilities report having positive life experiences, roughly two-thirds of Down syndrome pregnancies are terminated in the US.[189, 190] Surprisingly, it appears that health professionals are responsible for much of the apparent bias against children with disabilities.[191, 192] In a survey of healthcare professionals in the labor and delivery setting, 90 percent of respondents would be willing to terminate their own pregnancy (or that of their spouse) for a prenatal diagnosis of trisomy 21, trisomy 18, cleft lip and palate, Turner syndrome, or hypoplastic left heart syndrome.[192] Survey respondents included obstetric and pediatric residents and nurses, from both the labor and delivery and neonatal intensive care units.[192] Ten percent of respondents would refuse termination under *any* circumstances; however, among those who would, respondents were more likely to do so for a diagnosis of trisomy 18 and were less likely to do so for a diagnosis of cleft lip and palate.[192] Thus, children with disabilities (and their caregivers) appear to have very different perceptions regarding life with a disability than many healthcare professionals.

Compassionate care. In rare circumstances, infants born with life-limiting birth defects, i.e., conditions associated with [certain] death, may, after reasonable life-saving attempts, be offered "compassionate care," otherwise known as a "natural death." In such cases, the medical team provides "comfort care" while allowing the child to pass away *without* the support of medical technology. If there is no hope of survival, or of a meaningful existence, then prolonging intensive care, such as mechanical ventilation, is generally viewed by most reasonable people (including myself) as an act of "futility." Note, however, that allowing a "natural death" for a child who has a life-limiting condition is ethically quite different from offering non-resuscitation (euthanasia) for a disabled newborn who has a reasonable hope for a meaningful life. Such is the case for numerous birth defects and anomalies, including Trisomy 21, Turner syndrome, and hypoplastic left heart syndrome. Decision-making regarding infants with trisomy 13 and 18 is more complicated, as for many years these conditions were deemed "incompatible with life" (i.e., lethal anomalies). However, this is no longer true, especially among those *without* severe cardiac, pulmonary, or airway disease.

Trisomy 13 and 18. While mortality in the first month of life is as high as 32%, a recent European multi-registry study of infants with trisomy 13 and 18 found that infants who survived the first 4 weeks were likely to survive as long as 10 years.[193] This means that children with trisomy 13 and 18 can live much longer than previously thought, especially if provided with proactive medical support after delivery. Moreover, those with surgically-corrected heart defects are now living much longer than previously reported.[194] It is my view, then, that families who desire *proactive care* for an infant born with trisomy 13 or 18 should be provided this support without coercion or judgement.[195] That said, infants with trisomy 13 or 18 who either have complex heart disease or require pre-operative mechanical ventilation for stabilization are at a much higher risk of death, and may not be good candidates for surgical correction.[196] Thus, each child should be treated as an individual, and the goals of care should be addressed with sensitivity.[197] Unfortunately, some physicians and hospitals take a different view, so if prenatal testing suggests that you will deliver an infant with trisomy 13 or 18, and you share my views, then careful selection of your birth hospital is important.

Disabilities and meaningful work. A growing number of businesses are now employing physically and intellectually disabled workers—even in the for-profit sector, including Fortune 500 companies (See "top disability employers" on Monster.com). Bitty and Beau's (bittyandbeaus.com) is an example of a popular coffee company based in North Carolina that employs young adults with intellectual and developmental disabilities. By routinely hiring young adults with intellectual disabilities, Bitty and Beau's demonstrates that young adults with special needs can find satisfaction, meaning, and purpose, even in the retail sector. According to Ben and Amy Wright, the founders/owners, "When you value people, accepting and including them comes naturally." Thus, if societal views regarding children with disabilities are based on the perception that these children have a poor quality of life, that perception, too, is flawed.[184, 186]

Children with disabilities frequently have positive life experiences and find meaning and purpose in both social relationships and the workforce. Children with disabilities also bring joy to those around them and have a positive impact on the family and society. If your child is diagnosed with a physical or intellectual disability, or a "birth defect," then you are not alone. Likewise, if your baby is born prematurely or physiologically depressed (low Apgar score), conditions associated with cognitive or motor delay, then you are in good company. There is probably someone in your neighborhood, church, or workplace caring for a child with a congenital or acquired disability. We are better as a society for having these special children with us, and how we view and treat them says a lot about who we are as members of humanity.

So why discuss quality of life and the prevalence of disabilities in the population? To begin, disabilities come in all shapes and sizes, many of which are minor and go entirely unnoticed by the casual observer. Further, disabilities are much more common than you might expect. Developmental and behavioral disabilities is more common among infants born preterm, but only 6.3% of moderate to late preterm infants, the largest group of preterm infants, have mostly mild disabilities at age 2 years.[181] My advice, then, is to be cautious with pessimistic predictions regarding pregnancy outcomes of infants that are expected to have birth defects or disabilities. Remember, also, that the physician providing prenatal counselling may bring a very different ethical framework to these discussions. While it is true that infants with severe disabilities may face lifelong health-related challenges, and some have developmental and/or behavioral challenges, children with disabilities frequently live long, meaningful, and productive lives.

Finally, if you find yourself the parent of a disabled newborn—mild, moderate, or severe—then be encouraged. You may face challenges, but things are not as bad as they may seem, and numerous public and private support programs are available to support you. A growing number of public, social, and religious support groups are available to provide support and encouragement. The Americans with Disabilities Act (ADA), enacted in 1990, provides the legal framework for an extensive system of public resources developed to ensure that children with special needs are integrated into society. The internet is overrun with information for parents and caregivers. A simple search for "children with intellectual disabilities" or "children with disabilities" in your state or county will provide all that is needed to get started.

CHAPTER 11. CHILDHOOD VACCINES

Vaccine Safety and the Implications of Vaccine Avoidance

Conversations about vaccines have been among the most challenging of my career and perhaps my least favorite part of general pediatrics. Truth be known, these conversations were among the reasons I chose to leave general pediatrics and pursue subspecialty training in neonatology. Despite my natural aversion to the topic, I felt compelled to include this section as a topic of importance to the care of newborns.[198-200] Evidence regarding the benefits and potential complications of vaccines is conflicting, so it was difficult to balance competing views, but it was even more difficult to overlook the bias that was present on both sides of this issue. Overall, however, my interpretation of the scientific evidence is that arguments opposing vaccines are based largely on theoretical concerns and anecdotal reports, while evidence favoring vaccines is based largely on published epidemiologic research. We will examine some of the evidence here for your benefit.

> My interpretation of the evidence is that arguments opposing vaccines are based primarily on theoretical concerns.

Vaccines are safe for the vast majority of children. Unfortunately, there is some evidence that a *small number* of children are at increased risk of an adverse outcome following vaccine exposure.[201] For this reason, I do not dismiss the concerns of families who claim that their child suffered following a vaccine exposure. Nor do I dismiss the concerns of parents who fear *potential* harm from a vaccine exposure. It is a parent's prerogative to advocate for the safety of their child, and no institution, governing body, or agency should interfere with parents' rights to informed consent (more on this later). Notwithstanding my empathy for families such as these, and my endorsement of parents' rights, my interpretation of the medical evidence is that vaccines are safe and effective for the *vast majority of children*. One of my aims in this section is to support this claim with a concise review of the evidence.

Anecdotal reports of developmental delays. Despite a growing body of evidence that vaccines are safe, vaccine refusal continues to rise in developed countries worldwide.[202] Emotional accounts of parents whose children were "normal" before vaccine exposure and later suffered developmental delays (or regression) are hard to ignore.[203] Reports like this are rare when compared to the large number of vaccine successes, but nonetheless genuine and heartwrenching. The vast majority of these reports suggest that developmental regression was causally linked with the vaccine simply because the exposure (vaccine) preceded the outcome (developmental regression). The problem with this assertion is that it does not *necessarily* prove that the outcome was causally related to the exposure. Let me illustrate my point using the well-known relationship between cigarettes, matches, and cancer development.

> The association of an exposure with a subsequent outcome does not prove that the outcome is causally related to the exposure.

Association is not causation. Individuals who smoke cigarettes often carry matches, and indeed it is true that individuals who smoke cigarettes are more likely to develop cancer. However, carrying matches does not increase one's risk of developing cancer—smoking does. Thus, the undeniable association between matches and cancer development does not prove that matches are causally related to cancer development. In the same way, the fact that vaccines almost universally precede developmental delays (or regression) does not necessarily prove that developmental adversities are causally related to vaccines. There are numerous possible explanations for the onset of developmental delays (or regression), but the bias favoring vaccines is so strong that other possible explanations remain unexplored. If vaccines are not *necessarily* associated with developmental impairments, then how does one explain what is observed in the small subset of children who have impairments after being exposed to vaccines? The following is my attempt to explore several possible explanations.

Vaccines and developmental milestones. To begin, "normal" development is subjective, and this is especially true with regard to *early* milestones. As discussed in chapter 3, milestones are *functional*

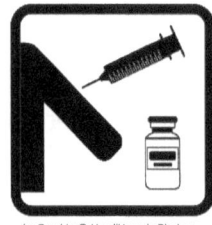

achievements (skills) documented at discrete ages (in months and years) that reflect a child's developmental progress over time. In otherwise healthy children, the first two years of life are characterized by a rapid but steady attainment of developmental milestones. Milestones are fairly predictable and provide meaningful insights into a child's developmental status and trajectory. Whereas developmental impairments are recognized when a child fails to acquire one or more anticipated milestones, developmental regression is noted when previously attained milestones are subsequently lost. Consider, then, that vaccines are administered early in the first year of life, when cognitive, language, and motor skills are relatively immature or evolving with exposure to the family and social environment. Thus, failure to attain milestones may not be appreciated until much later—sometimes as late as the second year of life.

The reality, then, is that vaccines precede the recognition of developmental delay or regression nearly 100 percent of the time because vaccines are administered, almost universally, in the first few months of life—well before most milestones are attained. Since vaccines precede virtually every subsequent outcome in childhood, then using the logic of most anti-vaccine proponents, vaccines could be implicated in the development of every adverse outcome in childhood! It should be clear, then, that this is not a rational argument. To be fair, other potentially dangerous exposures should be considered in the evaluation of infants and children with developmental delays, including genetic predisposition, naturally acquired infections, prematurity, and a host of chemical and environmental exposures too numerous to count in a volume as brief as this.

> "Normal" is always subjective, but this is especially true when it comes to the spectrum of early developmental milestones.

Vaccine encephalopathy. Researchers and physicians are generally in agreement that vaccine-related developmental delays (or regression) are typically preceded by a clinical syndrome called *vaccine encephalopathy.* There is no perfect definition, but *vaccine encephalopathy* is characterized by an acute alteration in mental status, including poor feeding, nausea, vomiting, lethargy (not awakening to feed), irritability, a high-pitched cry, and body stiffness or rigidity.[204] While vaccine encephalopathy is rare, it is generally noted within seven to ten days of vaccine exposure, but the adverse effects may not be recognized for months, perhaps longer. Herein lies the most important challenge for vaccine researchers—the exposure (vaccine) often precedes the outcome by many months, perhaps longer. Thus, the link between vaccine exposure and abnormal development is best established by documenting a period of *encephalopathy* within seven to ten days of the vaccine exposure. This is important, as anecdotal reports of an association between vaccine exposure and developmental delay (or regression) frequently lack this important association. The question might be asked, then: Is it possible for a vaccine exposure to be associated with developmental delay (or regression) *without* documentation of an acute encephalopathy? The answer is complex, but a brief review of vaccine history may be helpful.

The whole-cell DPT vaccine. Due to growing concerns about the *whole-cell* DPT vaccine in the early 1990s, a 10-year follow-up study to the National Childhood Encephalopathy Study (NCES, United Kingdom) was published in 1993.[205, 206] The study found that children who experienced an acute encephalopathy (a maximum of one case in every 100,000 DPT vaccines) within seven days of the vaccine were at no greater risk of chronic (permanent) neurologic dysfunction than children who had not received the vaccine. This prompted the US Public Health Service to convene a congressional committee study of the NCES report. Although the committee's initial findings did not support a relationship between the whole-cell DPT vaccine and childhood encephalopathy, the committee later reconvened and concluded that while there was insufficient evidence for a *causal link* between the *whole-cell* DPT vaccine and chronic neurologic dysfunction in children, it was *possible*, in rare cases (up to 10 cases per million DPT vaccines), that a chronic neurologic dysfunction could develop, even in the *absence* of an *acute encephalopathy*. The committee also suggested that the *whole-cell* DPT vaccine could (potentially) be a trigger for chronic neurologic dysfunction in children with an underlying predisposition to neurologic injury.

> The simple fact that a vaccine precedes the development of neurocognitive deficits does not prove that vaccines are causally related to neurologic injury.

Based on this and other evidence, the American Academy of Pediatrics recommended discontinuation of the *whole-cell* DTP vaccine in 1996, and by the early 2000s toxic bacterial metabolites were discovered in several *whole-cell* DTP vaccine lots, providing some explanation for the neurologic adversities noted in previous reports.[207] The whole-cell diphtheria, tetanus, and pertussis (DTP) vaccine was eventually removed from the market, and in 2018 an analysis of the Vaccine Adverse Event Reporting System (admittedly not a perfect system) revealed a significant reduction in the number of adverse events associated with the new and improved *acellular* DTaP vaccine (diphtheria, tetanus, and acellular pertussis).[201] While the DTaP appeared to be less effective, it also appeared to be safe—an acceptable balancing measure for researchers, parents, and pediatricians alike.

Unfortunately, vaccine-related adversities are still being documented in a very small number of children. So, the question remains: Does the benefit of vaccines outweigh the risk? In my mind, from a public health perspective the answer is "yes"—the benefits of vaccines far outweigh the risks. Let me explain with a brief summary of several areas of the vaccine research.

The MMR vaccine, autism, and inflammatory bowel disease. As with the DTaP vaccine, there is a growing body of evidence that the measles, mumps, and rubella (MMR) vaccine is not associated with abnormal developmental outcomes.[208-214] Scandinavia, widely known for its high-quality population-based research, provides valuable insights into exposure/outcome relationships in medicine. In a population-based study of over 1.8 million Finnish children, researchers found no association between the MMR vaccine and either inflammatory bowel disease or autism.[213] Likewise, an analysis of over 1.2 million children found no relationship between vaccination and (1) autism or autism spectrum disorder, (2) autism and the MMR vaccine, and (3) autism and either thimerosal or mercury exposure.[214] So if research suggests that vaccines are not associated with developmental delay or regression, then how does one explain the apparent increase in developmental and behavioral outcomes over time?[202, 203]

The answer, once again, is complex, but there are several possible explanations. To begin, the rate of developmental and behavioral disabilities is on the rise in the United States. The rate of parent-reported disabilities increased from approximately 12.8 percent in 1997 to roughly 15.0 percent in 2008, and both autism and ADHD have increased significantly during this period.[3] To a generation of parents that are increasingly influenced by digital media, web-based anecdotal reports of vaccine failure are widespread, and to some families these reports are frightening. In addition, better diagnostic tools and screening methods are available—tools unavailable only 20 years ago. Moreover, diagnostic criteria have been incrementally refined, including the ability to accurately diagnose mild cognitive and behavioral disabilities. Finally, there has been a significant increase in both the awareness and availability of resources for treatment of children with disabilities, increasing the likelihood and number of applications for and use of these resources.[215]

Why might some children be more vulnerable than others. This might explain the growing concern among families, but why are some children more likely to have an adverse response to a vaccine than others? One explanation is that some are more susceptible (vulnerable) to biological and environmental exposures than others.[216-220] There is a growing body of evidence, for example, that some children are more genetically predisposed to neurologic adversity than others.[221, 222] For example, progressive childhood encephalopathy derives from a wide variety of exposures, including genetic/metabolic disorders, viral infections (encephalitis), and chemicals/environmental toxins.[204, 223, 224] A large-scale population-based study reported that the overall incidence of progressive childhood encephalopathy is roughly 0.6/1,000 live births, and roughly two-thirds of these (0.4/1,000) have their onset within the first month of life.[225] In a review of cases of acute encephalopathy reported to the immunization monitoring agency in Canada, 70 percent of cases had a *more likely alternate cause* than vaccine exposure.[226] This suggests that in Canada only 30 percent of cases of childhood encephalopathy could be reasonably attributed to vaccine exposure, based on the timing of vaccines (exposures) and outcomes (encephalopathy).

The reality is that the newborn brain is more vulnerable during critical phases of development than that of older children and adults.[227] As discussed in an earlier chapter, the brain grows rapidly in the first year, with ongoing synaptogenesis, pruning, and patterning for up to three years, perhaps longer.[26] Immune-mediated genetic modification (sometimes referred to as *epigenetic programming*) is one of the mechanisms by which infants develop brain disorders before and after delivery.[228] Further, evidence suggests that some infants are more vulnerable to infection, inflammation, or environmental exposures than others.[228] This might explain why some children exposed to naturally acquired viral infections (e.g., measles) develop encephalitis and subsequent brain injury, while others do not. Therefore, immune (e.g., autoimmune) mechanisms might explain the variance in outcomes. In other words, genetically inborn vulnerabilities might explain why some are at greater risk than others.

Genetic predisposition. One way of understanding the concept of genetic predisposition is to consider what I learned in medical school regarding the *Knudson hypothesis*, i.e., the two-hit theory of cancer development. The Knudson hypothesis suggests that both genetic and environmental influences contribute to the development of cancer. It theorizes that certain individuals have a genetic *predisposition* to cancer and are somehow at greater risk of developing cancer when exposed to a second cancerogenic exposure, whether genetic or environmental.[229] In this way, genetically predisposed (vulnerable) infants could be at greater risk of an adverse neurologic outcome when exposed to infection, inflammation, environmental toxins, or some other metabolic exposure, including vaccines. In 1977, Folstein and Rutter published their findings of a study of twin pairs, demonstrating a genetic link with autism.[230, 231] This finding has been confirmed by others and suggests that autism has a genetic link. Likewise, in 2006, cases of alleged *vaccine encephalopathy* were linked to mutations in genes controlling sodium channels (within cells).[232] This provided some evidence that certain individuals may be at greater risk of an adverse vaccine reaction (e.g., encephalopathy) than others.

Vaccine successes and failures. While the history of the whole-cell DTP vaccine is troubling, the history of vaccine development is one of success, overall. Like so many medical advancements, the story of vaccine development includes a long series of successes and failures. However, the successes have far outweighed the failures. Modern Americans have enjoyed the benefits of vaccines for several generations. Life without smallpox, polio, measles, congenital rubella syndrome, tetanus, and pertussis is now an entitlement. But this was not so only a hundred years ago. Childhood diseases have declined significantly since the early twentieth century—undoubtedly the result of public health efforts to immunize the population.[233] Measles, a devastating illness associated with both death and neurologic disability, decreased from approximately 894,000 cases in 1941 to approximately 1,200 cases in the year 2019.[233] During the last reported rubella outbreak, between 1964 and 1965, over 12 million people contracted the disease, roughly 11,000 women lost their babies, and about 21,000 babies acquired congenital rubella syndrome.[233] Now, only a handful of people acquire rubella in the US, largely during international travel. After implementation of national vaccine recommendations for 13 vaccine-preventable diseases, there was a greater than 92 percent decline in cases and a 99 percent decline in deaths from diseases related to diphtheria, mumps, pertussis, and tetanus.[234] Although there has been a resurgence of measles and pertussis in recent years, poliovirus and rubella viruses have been essentially eliminated in the US, and smallpox has been eradicated worldwide.[234]

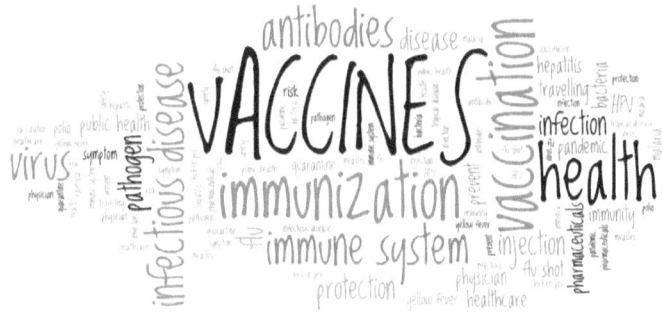

ID 103555009 © Tupungato | Dreamstime.com

Naturally acquired infection. Consider also that the risk of an adverse outcome is far greater after exposure to naturally acquired (wild type) diseases. Roughly one to two cases out of every 1,000 *naturally acquired* measles exposures results in encephalitis/encephalopathy, while only one case in a million MMR vaccine exposures results in encephalopathy.[233]

Admittedly, even one case of vaccine-related encephalopathy is tragic, but the risk associated with naturally acquired infection is far *greater* than the risk associated with the vaccine, especially in the context of increasing vaccine avoidance! While it is true that herd immunity (immunity related to vaccination of the population) has increased, and the risk of a wild-type exposure is far less than the risk in previous generations, the most important argument against vaccine avoidance is that very few vaccinated children have adverse reactions! So this is my first challenge for those who oppose childhood vaccines: if vaccines are so bad, then why have so few children had adverse consequences? Yes—vaccines are accompanied by a very small risk of long-term adversity, but only in a very small subset of children.[200]

Informed parental consent. Nonetheless, it is my strong conviction that parents should be informed of (and accept) these risks before children are vaccinated. Given the small but potential risk of long-term consequences, parents have the right to refuse vaccination of their children. Because vaccine refusal is accompanied by a significant increase in the risk of childhood diseases, some of which can be life-threatening and neurologically devastating, the risk of vaccine refusal should be clearly disclosed to parents, with impunity. Healthcare decisions belong to parents, not government agencies, educational boards, or pediatricians! Regardless of how compelling the argument or how serious the public interest, parents are the agents most qualified (and suitable) to make decisions for their children, especially when there is a potential risk involved.

One of the fundamental tenets of healthcare (and research) is the concept of *informed consent.* Pediatricians provide care to their patients under the umbrella of *informed parental consent.* So, what, exactly, does this mean? Informed consent is an individual's right to be informed of the risks and potential consequences of a proposed intervention or treatment. Implicit in this right, then, is the right to refuse! With regard to children, specifically, informed consent refers to a *parent's right* to be informed of the risks and potential consequences, and with this, the right to refuse. When reasoned, well-intentioned parents lose the right to consent, then the government, educational board, or its agents/liaisons have become dangerously intrusive!

Final thoughts on vaccines. In closing, I urge prospective parents to be cautious of anecdotal accounts that lack scientific rigor. Likewise, I urge health departments, government agencies, and pediatricians to disclose the potential risks and consequences of any proposed vaccine and to honor every parent's right to choose what is best for their child. In the wake of the COVID-19 pandemic, the American College of Pediatricians (ACPeds) issued an important position statement regarding vaccine development and vaccine mandates. Specifically, the ACPeds advocates for the development of vaccines devoid of any reliance on abortion-derived fetal cell lines. The rapid development of these and other vaccines has raised concerns regarding the utilization of cell lines that create an ethical dilemma for families (including mine). Assurances regarding ethical vaccine development are just as important as safety and efficacy. Indeed, at least two vaccine manufacturers have claimed that fetal cell lines were not used in the development of COVID-19 vaccine products. These assurances are crucial as we move into the era of transparent, family-centered care. Vaccine manufacturers, public policy agencies, and medical societies owe this to the citizens of a free, just, and benevolent society. Just as researchers must commit to the humane treatment of human and animal research subjects, so too must these agencies commit to ethical standards in the development and deployment of vaccines.

Finally, if you or your pediatrician have reason to believe that your child may be at increased risk related to vaccine exposure, whether real or perceived, then it is reasonable to consider a *modified vaccine schedule,* as proposed by others. It is my personal view that a modified vaccine schedule is far better than vaccine avoidance and a reasonable alternative for families who are concerned about the risks of vaccine exposure. The specifics of the modified vaccine schedule are beyond the scope of this book, so I leave this to you and your pediatrician. Lastly, I recommend a balanced view, one that acknowledges both the risks and benefits of vaccines—and one that considers the weight of the evidence.

CONCLUSION: PREPARING FOR THE JOURNEY

Thank you for reading my book; I am genuinely honored and hope you found it helpful. Recognizing the challenges of the newborn period is an important part of the parenting journey. But if you have read this book, and retained these concepts, you should be well-prepared for the challenges that lie ahead. It is my hope that your preparation has earned you a more enjoyable journey – the kind of enjoyment that comes with thoughtful care and preparation. In these final paragraphs, I offer a brief review of the most important concepts and conclude with suggestions on equipment and supplies that you may find helpful.

Research has shown that the home environment and mother-infant interactions, including human touch, can influence newborn development. A safe, warm, developmentally appropriate home environment is essential. Skin-to-skin care, for example, is associated with improvements in the initiation of lactation, breastfeeding success, and blood sugar stability. The most common complications of the early postnatal period are respiratory distress, early-onset infection, low blood sugar, and jaundice. While birth trauma can and does occur, it is generally unavoidable when it happens and is often the result of the obstetrician's attempt to minimize the risk of birth asphyxia or brain injury. Therefore, it is important to recognize that bumps and bruises, even fractured limbs, are relatively unimportant when compared with a healthy newborn brain.

Most newborns are born at a full-term gestational age, with a normal birth weight, and have all the usual signs of well-being. However, as many as 10 to 12 percent of live-born infants are premature, with a slight increase in the risk of adversity, including mild developmental impairments. Like prematurity, chromosomal abnormalities are largely unavoidable. However, infection is a potentially preventable complication of the newborn period, and several public policy efforts have become standard of care to minimize these risks. Fortunately, newborns have fairly predictable and recognizable signs of well-being, and the ability to recognize changes in the signs of well-being is fundamental to newborn care. For example, changes in appetite, behavior, or activity are important clues that a newborn may be developing an acute illness. Sick newborns typically present with one or more of the following signs of illness: poor appetite, decreased activity (lethargy), irritability, or an abnormal temperature ($\leq$ 97.7°F or $\geq$ 99.5°F). Any one of these signs of illness should prompt an immediate evaluation.

Some of the most serious signs of illness appear in appendix A, with an important disclaimer—the information provided here is presented as a handbook for your journey; it is not intended to replace your pediatrician. If temperature instability (high or low), lethargy, respiratory distress, or changes in skin color are noted, please call your pediatrician. All newborns have the occasional spit-up after meals, but vomiting that is either persistent, severe, or bile-stained (green in color) deserves a formal evaluation by a skilled pediatrician. Likewise, abdominal distension or persistent irritability could signal a serious illness. Any one of these signs of illness warrants an immediate evaluation by a physician or advanced practice provider. Pauses in breathing (apnea), seizure-like movements, or signs of dehydration should also be evaluated without delay. Colic is a diagnosis of exclusion, so other causes of irritability (inconsolable crying) should be ruled out before considering this diagnosis. However, like many conditions in the newborn period, colic is generally accompanied by many other signs of well-being. A good appetite is perhaps the most important of these, so a change in your baby's appetite could be a clue that something is wrong.

Infants born preterm and those with physical or developmental disabilities may require special attention from your medical team before hospital discharge, and generally require ongoing support from community service organizations. Nonetheless, most infants with physical or developmental disabilities live long, meaningful, and productive lives. Therefore, an optimistic view of the future is not only reasonable, it is also healthy, and supported by evidence. Healthcare workers may have a more pessimistic view of infants with disabilities, presumably because of the perception that children with disabilities (and their caregivers) have poor quality of life. However, evidence from the medical literature suggests that this perception is flawed, as quality of life ratings for children with disabilities are often similar to those of children and adults without physical and developmental disabilities.

Finally, developing a long-term partnership with a pediatrician is one of the most important investments you can make as you begin your parenting journey. While no pediatrician is perfect, there is no substitute for an experienced pediatrician who will listen and care about you and your newborn.

Well-baby visits serve two important purposes. First, these seemingly routine visits provide the pediatrician an opportunity to assess your newborn's overall health status. Is your baby eating well and gaining weight? Voiding and stooling regularly? Sleeping through the night by four months of age? These and other signs of well-being should be documented, and deviations addressed. Second, health maintenance visits provide an opportunity to evaluate your baby's developmental progress over time. The initial visit serves as a baseline and includes an assessment of baby's overall health and well-being, such as breastfeeding success, formula intake, feeding patterns, and sleep, among other things. Subsequent visits are compared with previous visits, and developmental milestones are documented at each age or stage of development.

The pediatrician is better able to provide guidance if he/she has had the benefit of observing your newborn's progress over time. While urgent care clinics provide an important service for pediatricians (especially after business hours), the physicians staffing these clinics are less likely to detect physical or developmental abnormalities than a pediatrician who has followed a child for weeks, months, or even years. On average, pediatricians examine between four and five thousand children each year, many of them newborns! With each visit, your baby enjoys the benefits of this experience. But there's more. The well-child visit also provides an opportunity for *anticipatory guidance*.

Gross and fine motor skills evolve rapidly in the first year, as do social skills and emotional attachments. At each age or stage of development, your pediatrician will provide guidance based on your baby's physical and developmental trajectory. Because each child is unique, the ability to recognize subtle differences in growth and development is essential. Which milestones are within an acceptable range, and which are not? Which findings deserve additional diagnostic testing or follow-up, and which deserve an immediate diagnostic evaluation? One of the most important reasons to invest in this partnership is that with each visit you gain the perspective of a physician who has learned to balance knowledge with experience and common sense.

The well-baby visit also affords your pediatrician an occasion for encouraging a safe and healthy home environment. When is it safe to take your baby out in public, to a restaurant, or to church? Is sunscreen safe? What about insect repellants? When is it safe to enroll your baby in day care, and what are the most important considerations for choosing a childcare facility? When can you safely introduce solids, finger foods, or whole milk? Which illnesses are going through the community, and what are the signs and symptoms? These and a thousand other questions are beyond the scope of this handbook, but are everyday questions for a pediatrician. A pediatrician's job is to provide just the right mix of common sense, experience, and knowledge, based on the best available evidence from the medical literature. By establishing a relationship of trust with a pediatrician, you are providing your newborn with the best chance for a healthy childhood. I recommend that you start establishing this important partnership on the first follow-up visit after hospital discharge.

Unfortunately, there is an exceedingly *small* risk of an adverse reaction to childhood vaccines, but a careful review of the medical literature suggests that for the *vast majority* of children, vaccines are safe and effective. Identifying at-risk infants is a true dilemma and perhaps the most important challenge for vaccine researchers, pediatricians, and public policy agencies of the future. Infants who are deemed at risk should be offered a modified vaccine schedule, which is far better than vaccine avoidance. Importantly, I am a strong proponent of the informed consent process, and by extension, a parent's right to refuse medical treatment. Whereas a parent's refusal to administer intravenous fluids to a severely dehydrated child would constitute parental neglect, the same could *not* be fairly said regarding parental refusal of vaccines or other potentially harmful medical treatments.

Equipment and supplies. One of the most practical ways that you can prepare for the arrival of your newborn is to ensure that your home or apartment is stocked with the supplies needed when the baby arrives. Consider placing small baskets stocked with newborn essentials at strategic locations around your home or apartment. Baby blankets, diapers, diaper creams, and other necessities can be stored in small wicker baskets or containers in convenient locations. Assign Dad the task of keeping these baskets fully stocked at all times. This gives your partner something meaningful to contribute while you are feeding and bonding with your baby. Stockpile as many diapers as possible, and by all means, allow your friends to contribute to the cause! One of the most creative traditions of the modern era is the advent of the *practical* baby shower. Raising a baby can be expensive, so allow your friends to defray the cost.

Other items to consider include a simple bulb suction apparatus for aspirating nasal and oral secretions, pacifiers, baby powder, petroleum jelly products, burp cloths, and perhaps one or two outfits as well. Petroleum jelly products are adequate for the mild diaper rash, but zinc oxide barrier creams/pastes may be needed for the angry rash. Believe it or not, the angry diaper rash can make for a *really* fussy baby. So it is far better to stay on the alert for wet or soiled diapers and keep

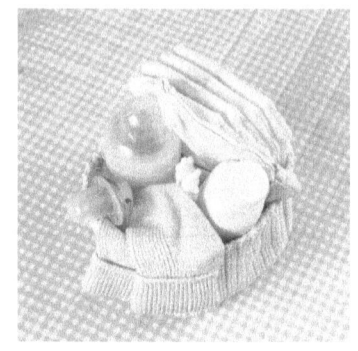

ID 179859647 © Anna Derzhina | Dreamstime.com

your baby clean and dry than to deal with the consequences. Most diaper creams and emollients provide a thin protective barrier from urine and stool (the offending agents). However, zinc aids in the healing process, so creams with added zinc facilitate healing. Baby powders are useful for maintaining dryness, especially in moist environments (skin folds, creases), but avoid powders that contain talc, as talc has been linked with cancer development later in life.[235] Baby powders containing cornstarch are widely available, and to my knowledge there is no known association between non-talc powders and cancer development.[236] Over-the-counter antifungal creams, such as clotrimazole, are helpful for treating mild yeast infections, but prescription-strength antifungal creams (nystatin) and oral agents (fluconazole) are available for the rash that fails to respond to over-the-counter remedies.

You can spend a fortune on baby products, so start with these basic supplies and save your money for the college fund! Consider keeping a good thermometer in the house as well. Digital thermometers are relatively inexpensive and easier to use than the mercury-filled type. Keep in mind that while axillary (armpit) temperatures and temperatures taken from the forehead are less accurate than oral and rectal temperatures, they are generally adequate. Acetaminophen (Tylenol) is another appropriate item for your medicine cabinet, but it is important to speak with your pediatrician (or pediatric triage nurse) before administering acetaminophen to a newborn. Acetaminophen can "mask" a fever and may make your baby feel much better. However, this can provide a false sense of reassurance when a baby is ill. It is important for your pediatrician to provide both guidance *and* follow-up for any treatments provided to your newborn, especially if your baby lacks the usual signs of well-being. Ibuprofen is generally prohibited in the first six months of life, so there is no need to have it in the house during the newborn period.

One of our favorite items, and one we considered indispensable, was the portable bassinette, better known in our home as the *Moses basket*. The portable bassinette allows you to keep your newborn nearby as you move around the house doing chores and activities. This simple item allows you the freedom to get other things done without being too far away from the baby and without interrupting the baby's sleep, which is important for a number of reasons we have already discussed. It can also double as a temporary crib for the first four to six months of life. The vast majority of cases of sudden unexpected infant death (SUID) occur in the first four months of life, and this is one of the reasons that pediatricians recommend keeping your newborn nearby during periods of sleep, especially in the first four months.

Newborns should sleep in the same room with their parents for the first four to six months after birth, but never in the same bed. Newborns are still gaining physiologic resilience (including physiologic brain maturation) for weeks to months after birth, and the portable bassinette allows you to be close enough to recognize the sometimes-subtle needs of your baby. Audio monitors serve a similar purpose, allowing you to be in a remote location but within hearing of your newborn's cry. You need not spend a fortune on these items as the baby will quickly outgrow the need for them. However, a portable bassinette and remote audio monitoring system are a perfect fit for your baby shower wish list!

One investment that my wife and I actually regretted was the so-called diaper disposal system. While the idea seemed good at the time, it was one of the more expensive items on our wish list and never seemed to deliver as promised. The general concept is that each diaper is deposited and sealed within a plastic scented film in a presumably airtight canister intended to minimize the lovely aromas that accompany the newborn period. Unfortunately, we were never able to avoid that odor. Indeed, our experience was that the strange combination of urine, stool, and scented plastic wrap seemed worse than the soiled diapers! Our diaper disposal system landed in the garage, largely unused. We opted for sealing each little gift in a leftover plastic grocery bag. To be sure, each diaper's tenure in the garbage bucket was short-lived, but our makeshift diaper disposal system served its purpose and was far less expensive! Now, don't get me wrong—the diaper disposal system may be right for you. You will find this and a thousand other items in the baby aisle of your grocery store, each promising a better newborn experience. As the father of seven children, I have spent lots of money on baby products over the years, many of which went unused. My best advice is to save as much as possible in the first few months; you have a lifetime to spend money on your children!

Family support. Let's face it, fathers play an essential role in the natural family and an incalculable role in raising children. Evidence suggests that both mother and baby benefit from a highly engaged father.[237, 238] In a study of over 1.3 million infants in Florida, mothers were more likely to have pregnancy complications and more likely to deliver preterm or low birth weight infants when fathers were absent during the pregnancy.[239] Other studies support this view as well, documenting the benefits of a highly engaged and loving father figure in the early stages of parenting.[237, 240, 241] Likewise, data from the Fragile Families and Child Wellbeing Study, which included over 2,700 unmarried mothers and fathers in 20 cities in the US, demonstrated that a poorly engaged or absent father during the pregnancy was associated with an increased risk of low birth weight.[242] The evidence favoring highly engaged fathers is so strong, in fact, that the absence of a father on birth certificates in Georgia was associated with an increased risk of infant death.[243] That said, if you have an atypical family, whatever that may look like, then a highly engaged and supportive partner or significant other may well provide many of the same benefits.

Maternal fatigue. The first few postpartum weeks are among the most challenging in the newborn period. Breastfeeding is especially demanding, as an already fatigued mother is expected to be available on demand, around the clock, for as long as two to four months. This leaves little time for uninterrupted rest, relaxation, or recovery. Maternal fatigue is common, and self-care becomes a distant memory! Without the support of an empathetic and willing partner, fatigue becomes routine and may lead to physical or emotional distress.[244] Postpartum depression affects as many as 15 percent of postpartum women, and while it is poorly understood, sleep deprivation and fatigue are contributing factors.[244] Postpartum depression has been linked with sleep disturbance and the absence of a regular routine, both of which have negative consequences for newborns.[18] In a study published in 2017, exclusive breastfeeding rates were lower among women with signs and symptoms of postpartum depression.[245] An actively engaged, loving, and supportive partner can make a huge impact on the health and well-being of mother and baby!

Selecting a pediatrician. A pediatrician or qualified family physician is an essential part of your support team. Grandparents, aunts and uncles, or even older siblings are key members of your family support team, but when the health and well-being of your baby are at stake, an experienced pediatrician is essential! Before starting my career in neonatology, I worked in a busy general pediatric office, examining between 25 and 35 children each day. In a typical year, pediatricians can examine as many as five thousand children, many of them newborns. Over the course of a career, a pediatrician can examine tens of thousands of newborns. So while Grandma, who raised six children and sixteen grandchildren, may have seen a variety of childhood ailments, your newborn benefits from the experience of a seasoned, objective physician.

Do your homework. Ask friends and family about their favorite pediatricians and select a pediatrician that works for you and your family. Most pediatricians provide an office visit free of charge before the delivery. Take advantage of this offer to get a sense of his/her practice philosophy and bedside manner. Pediatricians are generally busy and may examine as many as 40 patients in a single day. So set reasonable expectations for your visit, understanding that the best pediatricians often have a full waiting room! It is my personal view that bedside manner is less important than clinical experience. However, but you need to feel comfortable with your pediatrician, and bedside manner is part of the package. Bring a short list of the questions most important to you and select your pediatrician accordingly. Consider also that unless you are in a small community, most pediatricians share on-call responsibilities with other pediatricians, so you may as well get accustomed to the idea of seeing other physicians from time to time – a pediatrician who works 24/7 round the clock is an unhealthy pediatrician.

Well, that's all I have for you. Thank you for honoring me with your time and attention. I genuinely hope that your investment in *Newborn Essentials* is rewarded with a healthy dose of confidence regarding the well-being of your baby. Hopefully, your confidence will bring a more enjoyable introduction to your pilgrimage into parenthood. My advice is to take lots of photos, make many memories. and enjoy your journey through the newborn period!

Finally, if you found *Newborn Essentials* helpful, please visit my website, Newborn-Essentials.com, leave a brief comment, and sign up for periodic email updates related to newborn care!"

J. Wells Logan, MD
St. Johns, FL
JWLogan@Newborn-Essentials.com

PART III APPENDICES

APPENDIX A. CONDITIONS THAT WARRANT AN IMMEDIATE EVALUATION

Disclaimer—this section is provided as a brief medical reference for those who have specific concerns about their newborn. It is intended to supplement the medical advice provided by your pediatrician and should not be perceived as a replacement for a face-to-face history and physical examination. Please call your pediatrician (or pediatric after-hours support line) if you are concerned about your baby's health or well-being.

By now you should have a good sense of what I mean when I say that a baby has "all the usual signs of health and well-being." On occasion, the early signs of illness are obvious. Fever, lethargy, and acute-onset vomiting, for example, provide evidence of an acute illness, and these deserve an immediate evaluation by a skilled physician. Unfortunately, however, the signs of illness are sometimes more subtle than this, especially in newborns, and particularly in the initial stages of illness. A timely diagnosis is important for newborns, so here we explore *specific* signs of illness using the general signs of *well-being* as a framework for discussion. What clinical signs warrant an immediate evaluation, and what can wait until the next day? Here we explore these questions and provide relevant background for conditions encountered in the newborn period.

At some point in time, most newborns are exposed to any one of a number of viral and bacterial infections. Many of these pathogens are known as *fomites*, which means they can survive on hard surfaces, such as counter-tops and changing tables, for extended periods of times. Many viral exposures result in only mild symptoms such as nasal congestion, an occasional cough, or loose stools, but some are more serious. The early signs of infection are often subtle, so the absence of the signs of well-being should prompt a visit or call to your pediatrician. Fortunately, most mothers have a keen instinct when *something is wrong*. If your instinct tells you that something is wrong, listen carefully and act promptly! On the other hand, if your baby has all the usual signs of well-being, then there is no need to read this appendix—at least for now. Consider saving this for occasions when your baby is ill or has one of these specific signs of illness.

Poor feeding: decreased appetite

By now you should appreciate that appetite is one of the most important signs of well-being in the newborn period. This concept is so important, in fact, that it bears repeating. A newborn's appetite or ability to feed can be viewed as an important vital sign—the sixth vital sign. The absence of regular, vigorous feedings suggests that the newborn may be ill. While the occasional drop-off in feeding volume is probably okay, persistently poor feeding volumes suggest that something is amiss. When evaluating a newborn who presents to the hospital or emergency room with signs of illness, the first question I ask is: "How is your baby's appetite?" or "Has your baby's feeding pattern changed?" The remainder of the evaluation takes on an entirely different flavor if the feedings are not going well.

> A newborn's appetite is among the most important signs of well-being . . . a sixth vital sign.

On the other hand, the presence of a good appetite can be extremely reassuring, even in the context of other signs of illness. For example, a good appetite despite the presence of cold symptoms, such as a runny nose, cough, or congestion, suggests the newborn is probably okay. Depending on the combination of other signs and symptoms, observation and close follow-up may be needed, but the presence of a good appetite is nonetheless reassuring. Even in the *absence of fever*, poor feeding, lethargy, and irritability are among the most serious signs of an acute illness in the newborn period!

Abnormal skin color: the blue baby

Healthy newborns generally have a pink undertone to the skin, especially in the finger pads, palms and soles, lips, and tongue. Overall, the remainder of the body should have a pale/pink undertone as well. While African American newborns have darker pigmentation, they too have a pink undertone, especially in the finger pads, palms and soles, lips, and tongue. Therefore, any newborn with a blue or gray undertone should be evaluated by a physician without delay. Abnormal skin color may not be diagnostic of any single disorder, but it does signify one of several *serious* conditions. In recent years it has become the standard of care for newborns to undergo a pulse oximetry screen for critical congenital heart disease (CCHD screen) before discharge. However, not all critical heart diseases are detected by the CCHD screen. In fact, there is no perfect screening test, and the CCHD screen is no exception. Therefore, newborns with abnormal skin color, especially blue or gray skin, should be evaluated by a physician immediately.

Newborns with blue or gray color to the lips, tongue, or chest wall or a generalized gray skin undertone should be evaluated by a pediatric physician without delay.

Serious, life-threatening infections generally present with poor skin color. Fortunately, infants with serious infections typically have other signs of illness such as poor appetite, lethargy, irritability, vomiting, and dehydration. Abnormal skin color is so serious, in fact, that it is reasonable to consider it an exception to the general rule about the other signs of well-being. Remember, however, that mottling of the skin is fairly common, especially in cool environments, but mottling should resolve with bundling or increasing the environmental temperature. Nonetheless, changes in skin color as described here, especially if accompanied by signs of illness such as poor appetite, temperature instability, lethargy, or vomiting, warrant an immediate evaluation by a physician. As the newborn ages, fetal red blood cells (fetal hemoglobin) die off and are replaced by adult red blood cells (adult hemoglobin). This transition from fetal to adult hemoglobin is accompanied by a transient period of anemia that usually occurs between 8 and 12 weeks of age. During this period, the newborn may appear pale in comparison to the skin color at birth.

Labored breathing

Labored breathing. Abnormal (rapid or heavy) breathing is one of the most common problems encountered in the early postnatal period. Indeed, labored breathing is among the most common reasons for transfer to the NICU. Healthy newborns usually breathe comfortably at a rate of 25 to 45 breaths per minute, but occasionally as high as 60 breaths per minute when active. Rapid or labored breathing, especially if accompanied by chest wall retractions, grunting, or nasal flaring, deserves a formal evaluation by a physician. Indeed, any form of respiratory distress, whether it be rapid breathing (tachypnea) or chest wall retractions, deserves careful evaluation and follow-up in a hospital setting. Continuous pulse oximetry, which measures blood oxygen saturations, is appropriate. While labored breathing is typically associated with infections of the lower respiratory tract (lungs), so also are bloodstream infections and a variety of metabolic derangements beyond the scope of this discussion. Therefore, labored breathing suggests a high likelihood of an acute illness, which warrants an immediate evaluation.

The majority of respiratory infections encountered in the newborn period and early infancy are viral infections and have a self-limited course. Most viral infections in older infants and children are uncomplicated, but the newborn period is different. Consider that the upper and lower airways of infants are smaller in diameter than those of older infants and children and are adversely affected by mucus/secretions. Airway secretions decrease the effective diameter of the airway, worsening respiratory symptoms, so infants with respiratory illness may require supplemental oxygen or advanced respiratory support. For this reason, infants with signs of respiratory distress should be monitored in a hospital setting, where the appropriate support can be provided. Finally, because many bacterial pathogens are life-threatening and the diagnosis is not always clear, initiation of intravenous antibiotics is appropriate while awaiting the results of diagnostic screening tests.

Irritability: the fussy baby

The fussy baby is among the most challenging dilemmas faced by parents in the newborn period. Even normal, healthy newborns can cry for as much as two hours a day, and for things as minor as intestinal gas, a soiled diaper, or hunger! Keep in mind, however, that benign inconsequential irritability is relatively short-lived (one to two hours per day) and is generally accompanied by all the other signs of well-being—by now you should be an expert on this. With very few exceptions, healthy newborns are easily consoled, and this distinction is important. Three key differences, then, between uncomplicated, benign episodes of crying/irritability and episodes that warrant an immediate evaluation are: (1) the transient/short-lived nature of the episodes, (2) the presence of other signs of well-being, and (3) the ability of the caregiver to console the infant. Normal, healthy newborns may be fussy from time to time but generally return to baseline within a short period of time and are easily consolable. Colic is a unique exception, discussed at length in chapter 7, but newborns with benign irritability (and colic) still have a normal appetite, periods of quiet contentment, normal activity, and are *generally* easily consoled.

Newborns are generally content in the first hour or so after a feeding. However, swallowed air occasionally leads to gaseous distension and distress. Episodes of gaseous distension are often relieved by simply repositioning or burping the baby, but the "gassy baby" may benefit from over-the-counter simethicone drops (3 to 4 drops), which allows gas bubbles to coalesce and pass more readily. The severe diaper rash is another cause of pain or irritability. Diaper creams can provide a barrier between the skin and the offending agent, which is usually urine and stool. Changing the diaper, then, and treating any apparent diaper rash is a good start. Swaddling or bundling the baby, or simply putting the baby down for a nap, can also calm the fussy baby. However, the cause of irritability is not always apparent. The usual causes should be eliminated first, of course, before considering the more serious or concerning causes. If the usual measures fail to console your baby, or if the irritability persists for longer than three to four hours, a search for hidden sources of pain should begin.

> Deviations from baseline behavior, activity, or level of alertness may be an important clue that your baby is becoming ill.

Hair tourniquets around fingers or toes are uncommon but painful and easy to miss, as are corneal abrasions (a scratch or abrasion at the corneal surface of the eye). Hair tourniquets are identified by a careful inspection of each finger and toe. The corneal abrasion is difficult to diagnose but generally accompanied by excessive tearing and redness of the affected eye. Diagnosis of a corneal abrasion can be made in the pediatric office in a matter of minutes using fluorescein dye and either a cobalt blue or Wood's lamp. Each newborn is unique, so recognizing changes in patterns and behaviors is especially helpful in establishing a diagnosis. The most important determination is the presence (or absence) of the signs of well-being, as already discussed. In the absence of the usual signs of well-being, the fussy newborn should be evaluated by a pediatrician. The fussy newborn that continues to feed well, with periods of quiet contentment and adequate sleep, is probably just fine. However, the fussy newborn that presents with a poor appetite, especially if not comforted by the usual measures like a diaper change, bundling, swaddling, rocking, or feeding, should be evaluated by a physician.

Fever, low temperature: temperature instability

Fever is an important sign of infection. Indeed, fever during the newborn period is a cause for genuine concern, even in the absence of other signs of illness. However, a fever in the presence of other signs of illness, especially in the first few months after birth, should prompt a thorough evaluation by a physician. The normal temperature range for newborns (and older children) is between 97.7°F (36.5°C) and 99.5°F (37.5°C). While 99.5°F is the upper limit of this temperature range, environmental conditions, clothing, and activity can all impact a newborn's core body temperature. Therefore, a generally accepted threshold for fever is a temperature > 100.4°F (38.0°C) in the newborn period. Consider, however, that the acutely ill newborn is just as likely to present with a low body temperature (< 97.7°F). This, too, is cause for concern and should prompt a thorough evaluation by your pediatrician. Thus, in the newborn period both high and low temperatures are concerning for acute infection and should be brought to the attention of an experienced physician.

In healthy newborns, core body temperature regulation is maintained within a narrow range, whereas peripheral body temperature (i.e., the skin, limbs, and extremities) is less tightly regulated. Core body temperature is regulated by brain structures (the hypothalamus and autonomic nervous system) that control the dilatation and constriction of blood vessels in the extremities.[246] For example, axillary and skin temperatures are typically lower than both rectal (core body) and oral temperatures, and oral temperatures are slightly lower than rectal temperatures. Unfortunately, the newborn's ability to regulate core body temperature is poorly developed in the first days and weeks after birth. Therefore, temperature instability in the first few days may be related to incomplete maturation of these important brain functions.[247] In the first few days, a low temperature might simply be related to inadequate bundling or a cool environment—I recommend setting the thermostat between 71°F and 73°F. Regardless of environmental temperatures, temperature instability should always raise suspicion for an acute infection in the newborn period.

Hospital and community-acquired infections

Almost any infection poses a risk to your newborn, so even minor signs of illness deserve an evaluation for possible infection. As with many of the conditions we have discussed, the most important considerations are the same. Does the newborn have all the usual signs of well-being? Appetite, activity, and demeanor are the first things that should come to mind. Infection is generally accompanied by a poor appetite, temperature instability, or a change in activity in the newborn period, so the external signs of an acute illness often support the decision to seek pediatric care. Runny nose, cough, and nasal congestion are common signs of an acute viral infection. However, these are not necessary for the diagnosis of "suspected infection," as the signs of illness are often subtle in the newborn period.

Lethargy, vomiting, and poor skin color, especially blue (cyanotic) or gray skin color, are particularly ominous, regardless of other signs or symptoms. Changes in any one of these signs of well-being should prompt an immediate evaluation by your pediatric physician or provider. While many infections pose a significant risk to newborns, a comprehensive list of potentially dangerous infections is beyond the scope of this work. The following is a brief discussion of the *most common* community-acquired infections that pose a particular risk to newborns.

Bacterial infections. While bacterial infections in the newborn period are serious, they are also quite rare. Bloodstream infections, also known as bacteremia, sepsis, or septicemia, are associated with an increased risk of death in newborns. However, the likelihood of developing a bloodstream infection in the newborn period is more congruent with risk factors related to the pregnancy and delivery (i.e., within the first three days after birth).[107, 248] The overall risk of early-onset sepsis (within three days of birth) is between 0.3 and 0.5 infants per 1,000 live births, which is relatively high compared to infections acquired after the first three days (late-onset sepsis).[248] Further, late-onset sepsis is much more likely among infants with complications of prematurity and those requiring prolonged hospitalization.[249]

The two most common bacterial pathogens, group B streptococcus and *E. coli*, are generally acquired during passage through the birth canal or from contamination of the amniotic fluid before delivery.[107] In 2011, researchers published the results of a large outcome study and used this data to develop an *early-onset sepsis risk estimator*, which considers risk factors related to the pregnancy.[248] This tool is widely used by pediatricians to estimate the risk of early-onset infection relative to the general population. While bacterial infections are more amenable to treatment than viral infections, if left untreated they carry a much greater risk. Therefore, treatment of a suspected bacterial infection carries a certain level of urgency.

Viral infections. Viral infections are much less likely to occur in the first three days after birth but much more likely to occur in the context of social interactions within the community. The following is a succinct list of community-acquired viral infections that are associated with an increased risk to newborns in the weeks and months after birth.

Rhinovirus. Rhinovirus is among the most common viral infections encountered in humans. It typically presents with signs and symptoms of the common cold, including runny nose, cough, nasal congestion, and fever. Preterm infants appear to be at greater risk for hospitalization and other respiratory challenges in the first two years of life.[250] Like other respiratory viruses, rhinovirus is passed from person to person by respiratory droplets or after contact with surfaces (fomites) that harbor respiratory droplets. Strict handwashing and distancing are important for preventing transmission by symptomatic household contacts. The clinical spectrum ranges from mild/asymptomatic infection of the upper respiratory tract (a common cold) to severe/symptomatic infection of the lower respiratory tract (bronchiolitis), which is accompanied by respiratory distress in newborns. Other viral infections mimic the signs and symptoms of rhinovirus, including variants of coronavirus, respiratory syncytial virus, parainfluenza virus, and others. Some infants develop asthma-like symptoms, also referred to as *reactive airway disease*, which is accompanied by coughing, wheezing, and shortness of breath. Some but not all infants with reactive airway disease respond to bronchodilators such as inhaled albuterol. Infants with labored breathing should be hospitalized for monitoring of oxygen saturation levels, the possible need for oxygen, or higher levels of respiratory support.

Enterovirus. Like rhinovirus, enterovirus is a community-acquired viral infection that passes from person to person by respiratory droplets and fecal-oral transmission. Numerous genetic variants exist, so this virus is responsible for numerous childhood infections like hand, foot, and mouth disease, herpangina, and viral meningitis. Overall, enteroviruses cause mild, self-limited infections that resolve without complication. However, the newborn appears to be at greater risk than older infants and children, with serious, life-threatening complications occurring most commonly in the first week after birth.[251] Enterovirus is generally spread by contact with saliva, cough droplets, or accidental exposure to stool but also by contact with countertops or contaminated surfaces. Once again, strict handwashing and distancing are important for preventing transmission with symptomatic household contacts, especially in the first few weeks after birth. Like many viral and bacterial infections, the first exposure is far more serious than subsequent exposures. There is no specific treatment, but hospitalization is appropriate for symptomatic newborns, as many have poor oral intake, malaise, and vomiting and are therefore at risk for dehydration.

Respiratory syncytial virus (RSV). RSV is a common community-acquired infection and among the most common causes of the "common cold." RSV is typically accompanied by a runny nose, cough, and nasal congestion. Fever is variable, as with many viral infections, but temperature instability is especially common in the newborn period, as are apnea and respiratory distress, which increases the risk of hospitalization. RSV is primarily passed from person to person via aerosolized droplets. However, like many other viruses, it can be passed by contact with contaminated surfaces. Like rhinovirus, RSV may be accompanied by asthma-like symptoms or reactive airway disease, which resembles asthma. Some infants respond to inhaled bronchodilators (albuterol inhalers), while others may not, and some require hospitalization. Unfortunately, RSV can be life-threatening in the newborn period, especially among infants who develop apnea or low oxygen levels. Preterm infants appear to be at greater risk from complications, as are infants born with congenital heart disease; further, RSV appears to be a key determinate for the development of chronic respiratory disease.[252] Infants born at less than 28 weeks' gestation and those born with congenital heart disease generally qualify for Synagis, a monoclonal antibody to RSV, which has been shown to decrease the risk of hospitalization.[252]

Fifth disease. Fifth disease results from exposure to the virus *parvovirus B19*. Parvovirus B19 is a community-acquired virus that presents with a characteristic "slapped cheek" appearance to the face, fever, sore throat, headache, and in older children, a stomachache. Unfortunately, children exposed to parvovirus B19 can be asymptomatic for as long as seven to ten days, which means that affected individuals can expose others (especially pregnant women) to the disease without knowing it and long before the classic signs are recognized. This creates a challenge, as this virus poses a significant risk to pregnancy. Infection with parvovirus B19 in the first trimester increases the risk of fetal anemia and in severe cases, *fetal hydrops*.[253] Fetal hydrops is a rare but serious form of anemia that can lead to high-output heart failure and even death of the fetus or newborn. Pregnant women should avoid exposure to this virus, especially in the first or second trimester of pregnancy, and exposure to children suspected of having fifth disease should be brought to the attention of the obstetrician.

Influenza. While influenza is fairly uncommon in newborns, it is among the most serious viral infections encountered in children and adults. The signs and symptoms of influenza include fever, runny nose, cough, nasal congestion, and body aches. Secondary bacterial infections are more common among the young and old. Newborns, preterm infants, and those with chronic illness are especially vulnerable. The period of time between exposure to the virus and onset of signs and symptoms (the incubation period) varies widely and may be as long as four days, possibly longer. For this reason, family and friends may be asymptomatic in the early stages of the illness, thus exposing at-risk individuals. Individuals with influenza should be avoided for as long as five to seven days after resolution of signs and symptoms. Known exposures should be brought to the attention of your pediatrician as soon as possible. While there is no clear benefit to early treatment with oseltamivir or zanamivir (Tamiflu) in symptomatic individuals, its use in asymptomatic individuals (as a preventive measure) may decrease the likelihood of infection and *may* decrease the likelihood of transmitting the virus to household contacts.[254]

Pertussis (whooping cough). Like rhinovirus, enterovirus, RSV, and influenza, pertussis is transmitted by inhalation of airborne droplets, and usually results from exposure to individuals with a cough. One of the characteristic features of pertussis infection is the presence of a chronic, unremitting cough that persists well after other signs or symptoms have resolved. While much of the population has been vaccinated against pertussis, the pertussis vaccine is among the least effective vaccines on the market. That is, even among those vaccinated, the rate of successful immune protection is only about 85 percent, whereas most vaccines boast immune responses between 90 and 95 percent.[255] Further, pertussis is among the most serious infectious exposures during the newborn period. The clinical syndrome associated with pertussis infection is the *whooping cough*, which is accompanied by significant upper airway (tracheal) swelling and obstruction, which sometimes requires advanced respiratory support.

One of my most distinct memories as a young pediatrician was having to insert an endotracheal (airway) tube in an otherwise healthy infant with pertussis. Each of these illnesses is potentially life-threatening, and for this reason, each warrants a thorough evaluation by an experienced physician.

Coronavirus. Coronavirus is a common viral infection, and most strains result in a mild, uncomplicated course. While older children and adults are more vulnerable to severe illness from SARS-Cov-2, otherwise known as COVID-19 infection, data regarding its effects on newborns is limited. In a systematic review of 37 studies, including 364 pregnancies and 302 newborns, the majority of COVID-19 positive women were in their third trimester when presenting for care.[256] Of the 302 newborns in the sample, 65 (23.6%) were born prematurely, one was stillborn, and five (1.6%) were in critical condition after birth—two of these later died. Only 5 percent of the infants born to COVID-19 positive women subsequently tested positive for COVID-19.[256] However, emerging evidence suggests that young children are at greater risk of COVID-19 infection than initially predicted, especially infants and children affected by the delta variant. In a larger systematic review of the literature, which pooled data from multiple studies and included over 1,200 infants, roughly 50 percent of COVID-19 cases among children under five years of age were in infants (birth to 12 months); 57 percent were symptomatic, and roughly 7 percent required intensive care.[257] Overall, the available literature suggests that COVID-19 is less likely to affect newborns than older children and adults. However, it is nonetheless a serious disease, adversely affecting both pregnant women and newborns. Exercise caution during pregnancy, avoid exposure to potentially positive COVID-19 contacts, and *seek medical attention early* if infection is suspected.

Vomiting: gastrointestinal distress

Vomiting is a relatively nonspecific sign, and it is not always a sign of illness in the newborn period. As many as one-third to one-half of all newborns experience benign, uncomplicated vomiting, otherwise known as gastroesophageal reflux (GER). GER typically presents in the first days to weeks after birth and often resolves within the first six months. Only when accompanied by choking, poor weight gain, changes in skin color (cyanosis), or irritability does GER require treatment. As with so many other pediatric ailments, the clinical history is important, perhaps more important than the physical exam. It is helpful to keep a diary of possible exposures, as your pediatrician can read the "story" to rule out other, more serious causes of vomiting. Specifically, vomiting accompanied by acute changes in the usual signs of well-being (i.e., poor appetite, temperature instability, lethargy, or irritability) should prompt a thorough history and physical examination by an experienced pediatrician!

Several acute illnesses manifest with acute onset vomiting in the newborn period. Infection, intestinal obstruction, toxic ingestions, food allergy, heatstroke, and head trauma are just a few of the most serious causes of vomiting in the newborn period. Again, the nonspecific nature of vomiting suggests the importance of the clinical history to your pediatrician. When was the vomiting first noticed (onset)? How often does it occur (frequency)? And how severe are the symptoms (severity)? Is it accompanied by other signs of illness such as fever, lethargy, poor appetite, diarrhea, or bloody stools? Are signs of dehydration present such as decreased urine output or dry mucous membranes? The clinical history can provide important information as your pediatrician seeks to establish a diagnosis.

Green-colored (bilious) vomiting is a particularly ominous sign. Gastric secretions (juices produced by the stomach to aid the digestive process) are generally clear to yellow in color and have a sour (acidic) odor. Infants and young children with acute gastroenteritis "spit up" so frequently, and with such force, that gastric secretions are commonly noted in vomitus. While the distinction between bile-stained secretions and gastric secretions is challenging, the difference is quite important. Vomiting of bile-stained secretions suggests the possibility of an intestinal obstruction, which is a gastrointestinal emergency! Bilious (bile-stained) vomiting is a concerning sign, then, as intestinal obstruction is a potentially life-threatening condition requiring surgical intervention. Your pediatrician will understand the urgency of the matter and may initiate transfer to a children's hospital for evaluation. In the same way, vomiting associated with abdominal distension or bloody stools is concerning and warrants an immediate evaluation.

Abdominal distension: another sign of gastrointestinal distress

Abdominal distension is potentially a concerning sign of gastrointestinal distress. Consider, however, that most newborns have a slightly full but soft, rounded abdomen after a healthy meal—this is normal! A firm or rigid abdomen, or abdominal distension accompanied by tenderness to palpation, is concerning. Like vomiting, abdominal distension is a nonspecific sign, so the clinical history is important and other diagnostic tests may be needed to establish a diagnosis. Abdominal radiographs (x-rays) and/or contrast studies of the intestinal tract may well be needed. Importantly, abdominal distension accompanied by a poor appetite, bilious vomiting, or bloody stools should prompt a thorough evaluation by a physician or surgeon. The newborn period has its own unique set of gastrointestinal emergencies, including diverse types of intestinal obstruction, both anatomic and functional. These conditions are beyond the scope of this book, but abdominal distension, especially when accompanied by malaise and/or vomiting, is concerning for one of several abdominal emergencies and deserves an immediate evaluation.

Blood in the stool or diaper

Bright red blood in the stool. A grossly bloody stool is an ominous sign in the newborn period. Several gastrointestinal emergencies present with bloody stools, especially in the ill-appearing infant.[258] While the specific causes of acute gastrointestinal bleeding are beyond the scope of this discussion, grossly bloody stools should be evaluated by an experienced physician without delay. Remember, however, that blood-streaked stools (tiny amounts of blood) are often benign in nature, but substantial amounts of blood in the stool should be considered an emergency until proven otherwise.

Black, tarry stools. The presence of bleeding from the *upper* gastrointestinal tract (stomach or proximal intestines) usually manifests as black, tarry stools. Blood that passes from the upper gastrointestinal (GI) tract to the rectum has had sufficient time to be broken down by the intestines into its constituent products: *heme,* which is converted to bilirubin and causes jaundice, and *globin,* which is broken down into its protein precursors. Thus, as blood passes through the gastrointestinal tract, it changes in color from bright red to black. Thus, black, tarry stools suggest an upper gastrointestinal hemorrhage, which is generally a serious condition. Some infants have rather dark green stools, which should be distinguished from black, tarry stools. If there is uncertainty about the presence of blood, the stool can be tested for hidden (occult) blood using a reagent-mediated testing film called a *hemoccult* test. Regardless, your

> The most important elements of the history are no different from what we have already discussed. Does the baby have all the usual signs of well-being?

pediatrician can provide perspective and guidance regarding the diagnosis and management of bloody stools.

Diarrhea and/or dehydration

Gastrointestinal illness is relatively common in infancy and early childhood but can be especially challenging in the newborn. Because newborns with viral illness typically have a poor appetite, gastroenteritis places the newborn at significant risk of dehydration. For this reason, newborns (and infants) with excessive stooling or diarrhea should be monitored carefully for signs of dehydration. Newborns with more than 10 to 12 loose or watery stools per day should be evaluated without delay. In extreme cases, diarrhea can lead to hypovolemic shock! The earliest signs of dehydration are decreased urine output, a concentrated (dark yellow) urine, and irritability. Importantly, the dehydrated newborn is often unable to compensate for ongoing water losses. The oral mucous membranes become dry or tacky, the lips cracked, and the cry hoarse. In severe cases the heart rate increases and tenting of the skin becomes apparent. These are all late and concerning signs of dehydration, which if untreated can lead to shock. The dehydrated newborn is initially irritable but becomes increasingly lethargic with ongoing dehydration. Thus, newborns should be evaluated at the earliest signs of dehydration so that intravenous fluids can be administered. While older infants and children may recover from dehydration by taking small, frequent volumes of Pedialyte or Gatorade, this is almost *impossible* for the dehydrated newborn, and for this reason, hospital admission is appropriate. Your pediatrician will provide guidance.

Changes in urine output

As discussed, decreased urine output is among the earliest signs of acute dehydration and is generally related to either poor oral intake or excessive fluid losses (intestinal or urinary). Viral illness is probably the most common cause of dehydration in newborns, but regardless of the cause, any acute illness can lead to dehydration in the newborn. As we have discussed at length, acute illness is usually accompanied by poor intake and malaise, but some viral infections manifest with vomiting and loose stools or diarrhea, so newborns can become dehydrated quickly. Intravenous (IV) access is often needed to manage dehydration, as newborns are unable to follow instructions like older children and adults. Unfortunately, IV access is more challenging in the dehydrated newborn, as the veins, which are small to begin with, are even more fragile in the dehydrated state and can rupture during insertion of the IV catheter. For this reason, it is important to ensure your newborn receives appropriate and timely care. In other words, do not wait until your baby is severely dehydrated to seek medical attention! If your baby has signs or symptoms of dehydration, make haste to the clinic or hospital.

Excessive urinary output is extremely rare but is among the most common presentations for new-onset diabetes mellitus in *infancy*. If excessive urinary output is rare in the newborn period, it is only because diabetes is extremely rare in the newborn period. Urine output is unusually high compared to the child's baseline in new-onset diabetes, and parents often recognize the difference. Diapers are unusually frequent *and* heavy compared to typical diapers, and most parents notice this rather quickly. Nonetheless, infants with excessive urinary losses, dehydration, and/or fruity breath (a clinical sign of acidosis) should be evaluated for the possible diagnosis of infantile diabetes. Regardless of the cause, excessive urine output and/or weight loss, along with other signs of dehydration such as dry/tacky mucous membranes, tenting of the skin, or a hoarse cry, should be brought to the attention of your pediatrician immediately.

Persistent jaundice

While jaundice is common in the early newborn period, especially among breastfed newborns, jaundice beyond the first two to three weeks is unusual. The most common cause of persistent jaundice is "breastmilk jaundice." While there is some uncertainty, current thinking is that a substance present in breastmilk enhances intestinal resorption of bilirubin, thus leading to increased unconjugated (unmetabolized) bilirubin levels.[259] Another theory is that a substance in the breastmilk prevents the liver from converting bilirubin to its conjugated (nontoxic) form. Occasionally, breastmilk jaundice can last as long as six to eight weeks or more.[259] Other rare causes of persistent jaundice include abnormalities of the gallbladder and its ducts and abnormalities of thyroid function. Rarely, the *conjugated* form of bilirubin (bilirubin metabolized by the liver) becomes elevated, signifying a defect in bile secretion or metabolism; in this case referral to a gastrointestinal specialist is appropriate. While most cases of persistent jaundice can be managed without treatment, some require specialized care. In short, persistent jaundice (i.e., longer than three to four weeks) should be evaluated by your pediatrician.

Concerning rashes in the newborn period

Most rashes encountered in the newborn period are self-limited and benign, as discussed in a previous chapter. The few rashes that are of any consequence are so rare, in fact, that it seems unnecessary to discuss them here. However, rashes are so common in the newborn period that the most dangerous or concerning ones are included here for completeness. The rash that accompanies measles infection, for example, is rosy-red and splotchy in appearance, with small (1 to 3 mm), flat lesions that start at the face and hairline and spread toward the trunk and extremities. While measles infection resolves without consequence in most cases, on occasion it has serious, even long-term consequences. Since the introduction of the MMR vaccine, measles is extremely rare. However, outbreaks of measles still occur in the US, especially among unvaccinated populations, and may have serious developmental consequences.

Unfortunately, several other infections (mostly viral) present with a measles-like (morbilliform) rash, including rubella, parvovirus B19, enterovirus, and adenovirus. Rubella and parvovirus B19 pose a much greater risk to the developing fetus, especially in the first trimester. Enterovirus is a common viral pathogen that causes significant illness in newborns. Whereas adenovirus is less common, it too can cause a serious inflammatory response in newborns. With very few exceptions, the treatment for viral infections is supportive, so follow-up with your pediatrician is appropriate for infants presenting with a measles-like rash. Group A streptococcal infection (e.g., strep throat) is a *bacterial infection* that presents with a measles-like rash, but it is primarily an infection of school-aged children and far less common in the newborn period.[260] As with most serious infections in the newborn period, these infections typically present with temperature instability (low temperature or fever), irritability, lethargy, and poor appetite. Because of the serious nature of these infections, newborns presenting with a measles-like rash should be evaluated by a pediatrician without delay.

The only other concerning rash that arises with any frequency in the newborn period is the petechial rash. The petechial rash is best thought of as tiny pinpoint hemorrhages within the skin. The petechial rash results from either a low platelet count or an abnormality of the clotting cascade, either of which can be dangerous. What distinguishes the petechial rash from most others is that petechia do not blanch when pressure is applied. Most rashes blanch with palpation, followed by a brisk capillary refill (i.e., refilling of the capillary bed on relaxation of the pressure applied), but this is not so with the petechial rash. Unfortunately, platelet deficiency is relatively common in the early newborn period and especially common among infants born to women with preeclampsia or pregnancy-induced hypertension. Fortunately, platelet deficiency is usually diagnosed before discharge and typically resolves without treatment. If a petechial rash is noted on examination, however, your pediatrician will order a platelet count or complete blood count (CBC), which includes a platelet count, and review the maternal record for potential causes (e.g., preeclampsia). Several treatment options are available, including observation, but if the platelet count is low enough for treatment, or if the platelet count continues to decrease, your newborn should be transferred to a NICU for observation and management.

The floppy infant

Normal posture and tone are difficult to describe, but the floppy infant is often appreciated by even the casual observer. The floppy infant has a characteristic "frog-leg" posture, with the lower extremities *abducted* (away from the midline) at the hips and little to no resistance to passive range of motion during the physical exam. The arms may lie flat on the table, beside the torso, and may even be extended with little or no effort by the examiner. Newborns generally require at least some neck support in the first few weeks after birth. However, the floppy infant has significant *head lag* with the pull-to-sit maneuver. The floppy infant will slip through your hands when you attempt to hold him/her upright under the armpits and shoulders. Establishing a diagnosis for the floppy infant is complex, however, and includes consideration of both acute (infection) and chronic (neurologic) conditions, as well as rare inborn errors of metabolism, which are beyond the scope of this discussion. For these reasons, then, the floppy newborn should be evaluated by your pediatric provider (or a child neurologist) without delay.

Seizure-like activity and apnea

Seizures suggest the possibility of a serious brain abnormality, so seizure-like activity in the newborn period deserves an immediate evaluation by an experienced physician! Unfortunately, distinguishing true seizures from benign motor activity or behaviors can be challenging, especially in the newborn period. Even the seasoned pediatrician will proceed with caution in the investigation of a reported seizure or seizure-like event. Myoclonic jerks and other benign movements are common in infancy and easily confused with seizures. Myelination of the brain and peripheral nerves is incomplete in the newborn period, and this makes for unstable nerve conduction and "twitchy" motor movements. Sudden, isolated, and asymmetric twitches are common in the newborn period, especially when emerging from sleep. Likewise, normal, healthy newborns frequently have roving eye movements and non-sustained rhythmic movements of the eyes at the extremes of visual gaze. This is in contrast with the fixed horizontal deviation of the eyes (with or without rhythmic jerking) characteristic of *subtle seizures*. The challenge, then, is distinguishing true seizures from benign motor activity or muscle twitching, which are common in the newborn period, and a seasoned pediatrician can provide the perspective that only comes with experience.

Seizures are among the most challenging diagnoses in medical practice and generally have serious consequences if untreated. Unfortunately, seizures can have multiple presentations in the newborn period. Some are associated with rhythmic contractions and relaxations of the extremities (tonic-clonic activity), while others are associated with arching, extension, or posturing. Still others are accompanied by changes in neuromuscular tone or apnea (a pause in breathing for at least 20 seconds), which results in dangerously low oxygen levels, and deviations or twitching of the eyes and/or tongue. Most benign rhythmic movements of the extremities can be "settled" by applying steady pressure to the involved extremity. Rhythmic activity that persists despite the application of pressure is much more likely to be a genuine seizure. *Subtle seizures* are more difficult to diagnose, but any event accompanied by a change in breathing pattern or skin color (from pink to blue) should prompt an immediate evaluation for seizures. Whereas sucking or puckering of the lips is a normal newborn reflex, "lip-smacking" is one of the more common signs of subtle seizures in the newborn period. Finally, any event followed by a period of unresponsiveness or extreme sleepiness should be evaluated as a possible seizure.

The most common cause of true seizures in the newborn period is birth asphyxia (sometimes referred to as birth depression), as discussed in chapter 6, so pediatricians generally have a higher index of suspicion for seizures when evaluating infants who have a history of perinatal birth depression.[261] Is the seizure-like activity associated with a perinatal (around the time of birth) event, or was the birth uncomplicated? Is the event associated with other clinical findings, like apnea or color change? Does the event interfere with normal feeding and activity? If the answer to any or all of these questions is no, then the event is most likely benign and reassurance is appropriate. Nonetheless, even the suspicion of a possible seizure is sufficient to warrant a thorough review of the medical history and an evaluation by a pediatrician and/or pediatric neurologist.

Apnea. Apnea is a cessation (or pause) in breathing for 20 seconds or more. Apnea is often accompanied by other signs of illness, such as fever, lethargy, poor feeding, or poor color, but *apnea is always the result of a serious condition*. Apnea is commonly experienced by premature infants, especially those born at less than 34 weeks' gestation, and for this reason infants born at less than 34 weeks' gestation are routinely treated with caffeine, which stimulates the respiratory centers in the brain. However, apnea can also be observed in full-term infants. Newborns with either viral or bacterial infections are at greater risk of developing apnea, regardless of the gestational age at birth. Apnea can also be seen with seizures, low oxygen levels, low blood sugar, and low body temperature. Regardless of the cause, any pause in breathing lasting longer than 20 seconds or accompanied by a change in skin color (from pink to blue) warrants an immediate evaluation by a physician. It follows, then, that any newborn with apnea or a sudden change in color (central cyanosis) should be monitored in an intensive care setting (neonatal or pediatric intensive care unit) where appropriate treatments, including oxygen or mechanical ventilation, can be provided.

APPENDIX B. COMMON BIRTH DEFECTS AND PHYSICAL OR DEVELOPMENTAL DISABILITIES

Maternal exposure to pesticides, chemicals, alcohol, and tobacco during pregnancy have all been linked with congenital birth defects, and the risk of these exposures is greatest during the first trimester of pregnancy.[262] The prevalence of birth defects is also greater among infants born to women over 35 years of age.[263] Fortunately, some of these risk factors can be addressed, if only in part. For example, maternal obesity, diabetes, smoking, and inadequate folic acid intake are well-documented risk factors for birth defects, and each of these can be avoided to some degree.[263] While challenging, good prenatal care and a genuine commitment to a healthy pregnancy can mitigate at least *some* of these risks.

Poorly controlled diabetes is the most well-known cause of birth defects, and the likelihood of a major birth defect increases substantially among mothers with poorly controlled gestational or insulin-dependent diabetes.[264] The risk of congenital heart disease, for example, is significantly greater among pregnancies complicated by diabetes.[265] For this reason, a glucose tolerance test is an important component of your prenatal care. Regardless of the circumstances surrounding the diagnosis, diet and blood sugar control are essential for minimizing the risk of birth defects during pregnancy.

Roughly 3 percent of live births are affected by a major birth defect.[266] The most common of these are trisomy 21 (Down syndrome), cleft lip and/or palate, congenital heart defects (e.g., ventricular septal defect), neural tube defects (spina bifida), and intestinal atresias (intestinal discontinuity or obstruction).[267] Only rarely do birth defects present as a medical emergency in the newborn period. Micrognathia, a condition in which the lower jaw is small and the tongue is posteriorly rotated, is a condition that may affect a newborn's breathing just after birth. However, micrognathia is rare, and the vast majority of major birth defects are uncomplicated just after birth. While major birth defects are rare, they are nonetheless a great concern for parents and healthcare professionals, and perceptions regarding quality of life generally do not reflect the real-life experience of children with disabilities (and their families), as discussed in chapter 10.

Importantly, major birth defects are rare by comparison to minor birth defects and are much more likely to be accompanied by physical and developmental disabilities. The emphasis here is on minor birth defects, as roughly 12 to 14 percent of live-born infants will have at least one minor birth defect.[268] Minor birth defects tend to occur in isolation, and when seen in isolation are generally *not* accompanied by major birth defects or disabilities. However, as the number of minor anomalies increases, so also does the risk of a major defect.[268] For this reason, the presence of two or more minor defects should prompt a search for other birth defects. In such cases, your pediatrician may wish to order a kidney ultrasound, an echocardiogram (ultrasound of the heart), or other diagnostic tests, depending on the defect identified. Genetic testing, which generally requires a blood sample, may be appropriate as well. Fortunately, genetic testing has evolved rapidly in recent years, and genetic diagnoses can be established in a matter of days to weeks. A few of the most common minor birth defects are included in the paragraphs that follow.

Conditions affecting the eyes

Misalignment of the eyes (strabismus). Strabismus, which appears to the casual observer as a misalignment of the eyes (to some, "cross-eyed"), is generally related to weak eye muscles and among the most common eye conditions in the newborn period. Strabismus in the first month or so after birth is considered a normal, transient condition. However, if it persists beyond the first two to three months, referral to a pediatric ophthalmologist is warranted. If left untreated, strabismus can lead to amblyopia (lazy eye), a serious condition in which the brain neglects the image of the affected (nondominant) eye. There is now some evidence that strabismus is associated with maternal smoking—yet another reason to avoid smoking during pregnancy. In a study of over 4,800 children, maternal smoking was associated with strabismus, and the likelihood of childhood strabismus was greater among children whose mothers smoked more than 10 cigarettes per day.[144] However, strabismus is generally a transient condition that resolves within six to eight weeks of birth. Patching of the dominant eye and surgical correction by a pediatric ophthalmologist are available for complex or persistent cases, and these are generally associated with good long-term outcomes.[269]

Cloudy cornea. Cloudy cornea is one of the most serious eye conditions in the newborn period, appearing as a dull, hazy opacification of the clear anterior part of the eye. While rare, a cloudy cornea suggests the possibility of glaucoma, an elevation of the pressure within the globe of the affected eye.[270] Several congenital viral infections also present with a cloudy cornea, and while some are not amenable to treatment, some are, and prompt evaluation and treatment is important.[270] Regardless of the cause, cloudy cornea should be evaluated by a pediatric ophthalmologist as soon as possible, as delayed diagnosis can lead to poor outcomes.[270] The diagnosis may not be established immediately, as many newborns have swelling of the eyelids and surrounding tissues and examination of the eyes is difficult in the first day or two after birth, Fortunately, cloudy cornea is extremely rare and is usually apparent to even the casual observer.

Conditions affecting the ear, nose, mouth, and throat

Cleft lip and palate. While cleft lip and palate are considered major birth defects, they are included here because they are among the most common birth defects encountered in the US, with roughly 0.7 to 0.9 cases per 1,000 live births.[271] As with strabismus, maternal smoking in the first trimester has been implicated as a possible cause of cleft lip and palate.[272] Indeed, smoking during pregnancy is associated with preterm birth, low birth weight, and several birth defects, including cleft lip and palate. The challenges of cleft lip and palate are related primarily to feeding and nutrition. However, your pediatrician and nursery staff will have several strategies for feeding success when challenges arise. Upright feeding and feeding with the Haberman Feeder (or similar feeding systems) are designed to simulate breastfeeding, which involves a different mechanism for expelling milk than traditional feeding systems. Each baby is unique, however, so an experienced nurse or lactation specialist can be a valuable asset. Overall, infants with cleft lip and palate will grow and thrive with supportive feeding approaches until surgical correction can be performed later in the first year of life. Occasionally, surgeons will delay surgical correction to the second year, depending on the nature and severity of the defect and surgeon preference. Early referral to an oral and maxillofacial surgeon or an experienced pediatric head and neck surgeon is appropriate.

Laryngomalacia (floppy airway). Like anomalies of the nasopharynx, upper airway (windpipe) abnormalities typically present soon after birth with noisy breathing (stridor), which is more prominent during the inspiratory phase of the breathing cycle. Perhaps the most common of these is a condition called *laryngomalacia*. The term *laryngomalacia* means *floppy larynx*. The larynx is the part of the trachea that houses the vocal cords, or "voice box." The clinical spectrum of laryngomalacia ranges from mild to severe, but most newborns with laryngomalacia have mild, asymptomatic stridor, a high-pitched inspiratory noise that gets worse with activity or feeding. Milder forms tend to resolve with time as the cartilaginous tissues within the airway grow and become more rigid. However, infants with mild asymptomatic laryngomalacia are at greater risk of developing respiratory compromise with upper respiratory infections, including the common cold. Infants with *symptomatic* laryngomalacia can present with respiratory distress or low oxygen levels and should be transferred to a neonatal intensive care unit for evaluation and management.

Abnormalities of the external ear. While uncommon, *low-set ears* are generally recognized soon after delivery and suggest at least the possibility of other birth defects. Low-set ears are defined by the line extending along the top of the ear (pinna) falling below the horizontal plane connecting the outer corners of the eyes. In a research study published in 2018, roughly one-third of spontaneously aborted fetuses had low-set ears, and these had a wide range of end-organ anomalies.[273] Therefore, the presence of low-set ears should prompt an evaluation for other malformations or anomalies. Fortunately, the universal hearing screen is considered a standard of care in the US, so any hearing impairment should be detected by the hearing screen before discharge from the hospital. Regardless of the size, position, or shape of the ears, a failed hearing screen should prompt a formal hearing evaluation by an audiologist and ear, nose, and throat specialist.

Pre-auricular skin tags and pits. Pre-auricular skin tags are small pedunculated, skin-covered soft tissue nodules that protrude from the skin just anterior to the ear. Pre-auricular pits are found in the same location, just anterior to the ear, but present as a tiny, shallow pit. These, too, fall into the category of mild congenital anomalies and are associated with a slightly increased risk of hearing loss. In a study published in 2008, researchers evaluated the outcomes of over 68,000 newborns who participated in a universal hearing screen program over a period of seven years.[274] The rate of hearing impairment was roughly eight per 1,000 live births among infants with pre-auricular skin tags or pits and roughly 1.5 per 1,000 live births without them. Once again, the universal hearing screen is a more reliable way of identifying infants at risk for congenital hearing loss, but the presence of a pre-auricular pit or skin tag should prompt a more formal audiologic screening test, especially in the context of a failed hearing screen.

Conditions affecting the skin

Capillary hemangioma. Roughly 5 to 10 percent of all children are diagnosed with a capillary hemangioma within the first year of life.[275] A hemangioma is simply an overgrowth of vascular (blood vessel) tissue within the skin or soft tissues and the most common vascular anomaly in childhood. Roughly one-third of hemangiomas are visible at birth, but the majority become visible within four to six weeks, increasing in size over the following six to nine months.[275] Capillary (strawberry) hemangiomas are the most common type and are found at the skin surface, but involvement of the subcutaneous and deep soft tissues is also possible, including the liver, neck, face, and eye sockets (orbits). Subcutaneous hemangiomas are typically blue-to-purple in color, with a spongy consistency that may or may not be visible at the skin surface. Hemangiomas in the deep soft tissues are generally not visible but can become quite large, occasionally leading to high-output heart failure. Ultrasound (or MRI) imaging of the liver and kidneys is appropriate in the setting of multiple superficial or subcutaneous hemangiomas. Hemangiomas affecting the face, neck, or visual fields are rare, but when present require additional imaging of the head and neck. Consultation with a dermatologist or plastic surgeon is appropriate in the setting of multiple hemangiomas, and medical or surgical intervention may be needed for large hemangiomas or those affecting the neck or face.

Conditions affecting the extremities

Clinodactyly is a common, uncomplicated anomaly of the hands (and feet) seen in as many as 20 percent of all live births.[276] Clinodactyly is the medical term that describes a characteristic curvature of a finger (or toe) within the same plane as the palm of the hand (or foot), most commonly the fifth (smallest) digit of the hand or foot. The curvature is typically noted at the most distal joint of the finger (i.e., the joint closest to the fingertip). It is much more common in children with Down syndrome (and other trisomy syndromes), but the incidence varies because the literature lacks a precise definition of clinodactyly.[276] In isolation it is a benign condition and should not be a cause for great concern. In my humble opinion, this anomaly does not warrant intervention or referral to a specialist.

Polydactyly (extra digits of the hands and feet). Also known as *supernumerary* digits, polydactyly is seen in as many as one out of every 500 live births. While differences in race and gender have been reported, polydactyly is among the most common birth defects of the hands and feet. It is usually found in isolation with no long-term consequences.[277] However, if found in conjunction with other anomalies, genetic testing and/or consultation with a genetic specialist is appropriate. A supernumerary digit is a soft, floppy remnant of a finger (or thumb) that has little to no cartilaginous tissue. Often smaller than the neighboring finger (or toe), it is located lateral to the pinkie finger or medial (toward the midline) to the thumb and has a thin/rudimentary connection with the adjacent digit. Rarely, a cartilaginous connection with the neighboring digit may be present, and in this situation referral to a plastic surgeon is appropriate. Polydactyly tends to run in families but in isolation is not a cause for concern and does not warrant referral to a specialist.

Syndactyly is another common, benign birth defect of the hands and feet with a reported prevalence as high as one case in every 250 live births.[278, 279] The term syndactyly derives from a combination of the words *syn* (together) and *dactylos* (digit). It is simply a failure of the fingers to separate during gestation, giving the appearance of webbed fingers. Both familial inheritance and spontaneous genetic causes have been reported. Like other minor anomalies, syndactyly often presents in isolation, but it can also be seen in combination with other genetic disorders. When seen in the context of other minor anomalies, a search for other end-organ anomalies is appropriate.[279]

Metatarsus adductus (in-toeing). In-toeing is a benign condition in which the long bones of the forefoot (metatarsus bones) are deviated toward the midline (big toe). Metatarsus adductus is best thought of as a *deformation*, as it is typically caused by abnormal positioning (i.e., crowding) during gestation.[280]. With an incidence of roughly one in every 500 live births, it is one of the most common orthopedic conditions of the newborn period. While in-toeing is generally uncomplicated, some children will develop bunions later in life, but I can think of worse things than bunions.[281] In most cases, the deformity can be manually reduced (straightened), if only transiently. In clinical practice, the ability to manually straighten the forefoot *without causing pain or discomfort* confirms the diagnosis of uncomplicated in-toeing. Most cases resolve with weight-bearing by nine to twelve months of age.[282] Physical therapy or casting may be needed in moderate to severe cases, but surgical correction is rarely necessary.

Developmental dysplasia of the hip is a condition in which the socket of the hip is shallow and the ligaments that maintain hip positioning (within the hip socket) are loose, allowing the head of the femur (the upper part of the leg bone) to slip in and out of the socket easily. It is seen in roughly 1.3 out of every 1,000 live births, making it one of the most common orthopedic conditions of the newborn period.[283] In the short term, developmental dysplasia of the hip is not problematic. However, if diagnosis and treatment are delayed, the hip fails to develop normally. The cause of developmental hip dysplasia is probably related to several factors and includes pregnancy hormones intended to loosen maternal pelvic ligaments (in preparation for childbirth), thus loosening the ligaments in the newborn, and familial inheritance. However, newborn girls and infants who were in the breech position during pregnancy are at increased risk. While some consider developmental hip dysplasia a major birth defect, it is also fairly common and easily treated if identified in a timely manner. The diagnosis is typically made in the newborn nursery soon after birth when the pediatrician identifies a "click" or "clunk" during the physical examination of the hips.

Conditions affecting the heart

Ventricular septal defect (VSD) is a congenital heart defect involving the ventricular septum, which separates the two large pumping chambers of the heart—the left and right ventricles.[284] The defect allows blood to be shunted away from the systemic circulation (the brain and body) toward the lungs and pulmonary circulation, which can lead to over-circulation, or excess blood flow to the lungs. VSD is the most common congenital heart anomaly, seen in roughly two to three out of every 1,000 live births.[285] The outcome is generally quite good, but early identification is important as surgical correction by an experienced cardiothoracic surgeon is usually needed within the first six months of life. Unfortunately, VSD is generally not diagnosed in the first few days after birth because of the unique *transitional* physiology of the newborn period. The characteristic heart murmur is often discovered at one of the first follow-up visits (after discharge from the hospital) with your pediatrician. The most appropriate diagnostic test to evaluate a heart murmur is an echocardiogram. Some VSDs are small and close (with growth and nutrition) spontaneously. While small to moderate-sized VSDs may close spontaneously, if left uncorrected, a large VSD can lead to over-circulation or congestive heart failure. Moderate to large VSDs generally require surgical closure in the operating room or cardiac catheterization laboratory, usually between four and six months of age. Early referral to a pediatric cardiologist is appropriate.

Conditions affecting the kidney and urinary tract

Hydronephrosis (swelling of the kidney) is among the most common abnormalities identified on a prenatal (screening) ultrasound. Roughly one to four out of every 100 pregnancies result in a prenatal diagnosis of hydronephrosis. Hydronephrosis results from a variety of kidney abnormalities, but the majority are mild, resolving without treatment. Follow-up is extremely important, however, as in rare cases hydronephrosis signifies the *possibility* of a serious kidney disorder. Hydronephrosis is included here, in part because it is such a common finding on prenatal ultrasound, but also to emphasize the importance of appropriate follow-up. Even mild, uncomplicated cases of hydronephrosis require follow-up, as these infants are at greater risk of urinary tract infections and other complications of the urinary tract.[286] After delivery, a diagnostic kidney ultrasound should be obtained for reliable imaging of the kidneys, ureters (connective tubes), and bladder. Depending on ultrasound findings, additional testing or referral to a specialist (pediatric nephrologist or urologist) may be appropriate.

Hypospadias. Hypospadias is a birth defect unique to boys, as it involves the foreskin, glans, or shaft of the penis. Approximately six out of every 1,000 males are born with hypospadias, making it one of the most common birth defects in the US.[287] Known risk factors include infants born SGA, infants born to multiple gestation pregnancies, and premature birth, and about 20 percent of males born with hypospadias had one of these risk factors. The most common type of hypospadias is mild, in which the urethral opening exits at the head (glans) of the penis (sub-coronal hypospadias). Less commonly, the urethral opening is seen at the midshaft (midshaft hypospadias) or where the shaft and the scrotum meet (penoscrotal hypospadias). Regardless of the severity of hypospadias, your pediatrician should consult a pediatric urologist for assessment and possible surgical management. Because surgical correction may be needed, circumcision should be avoided until the urologist has had the opportunity to evaluate and make recommendations. A kidney ultrasound is usually obtained before discharge to rule out other abnormalities of the urinary tract.

Conditions affecting the back or spine

Tethered spinal cord. The lowermost, terminal end of the spinal cord is called the conus medullaris. Ordinarily, the spinal cord ends at the level of second or third lumbar spine, but occasionally the distal spinal cord becomes *tethered* (attached) to the surrounding tissues and is unable to move with growth/elongation of the spinal cord. This condition is seen in as few as one out of every 4,000 live births.[288] If unrecognized, however, it can lead to nerve damage as the spinal cord grows. Bowel and bladder dysfunction are among the more serious consequences, and difficulties with ambulation/walking can occur. Fortunately, a thorough physical examination during the newborn period can provide clues to the diagnosis. A raised bulge, a tuft of hair, a dimple, or an unusual discoloration at the lower end of the spine (near the gluteal cleft) can be seen in infants with an underlying tethered spinal cord. The good news is that while the consequences are serious, the injury occurs with growth over many months, which leaves your pediatrician plenty of time to establish a diagnosis and make an appropriate referral. A screening lumbosacral ultrasound at four to six weeks after birth is appropriate, but the diagnosis should be confirmed with an MRI of the lumbosacral spine. Referral to a pediatric neurosurgeon within the first four to six months is appropriate so that surgical correction can be performed before nerve damage occurs.

References

1.   Shapiro-Mendoza CK, Lackritz EM. Epidemiology of late and moderate preterm birth. Semin Fetal Neonatal Med. 2012;17(3):120-5.
2.   Moon RY, Hauck FR. SIDS Risk: It's More Than Just the Sleep Environment. Pediatrics. 2016;137(1).
3.   Boyle CA, Boulet S, Schieve LA, Cohen RA, Blumberg SJ, Yeargin-Allsopp M, et al. Trends in the prevalence of developmental disabilities in US children, 1997-2008. Pediatrics. 2011;127(6):1034-42.
4.   Mai CT, Isenburg JL, Canfield MA, Meyer RE, Correa A, Alverson CJ, et al. National population-based estimates for major birth defects, 2010-2014. Birth Defects Res. 2019;111(18):1420-35.
5.   Ronfani L, Vecchi Brumatti L, Mariuz M, Tognin V, Bin M, Ferluga V, et al. The Complex Interaction between Home Environment, Socioeconomic Status, Maternal IQ and Early Child Neurocognitive Development: A Multivariate Analysis of Data Collected in a Newborn Cohort Study. PLoS One. 2015;10(5):e0127052.
6.   Gualdron LMV, Villalobos MMD. Effect of infant stimulation on the adaptation to birth: a randomized trial. Rev Lat Am Enfermagem. 2019;27:e3176.
7.   Ornoy A. The impact of intrauterine exposure versus postnatal environment in neurodevelopmental toxicity: long-term neurobehavioral studies in children at risk for developmental disorders. Toxicol Lett. 2003;140-141:171-81.
8.   Kanto WP, Jr., Calvert LJ. Thermoregulation of the newborn. Am Fam Physician. 1977;16(5):157-63.
9.   Azaz Y, Fleming PJ, Levine M, McCabe R, Stewart A, Johnson P. The relationship between environmental temperature, metabolic rate, sleep state, and evaporative water loss in infants from birth to three months. Pediatr Res. 1992;32(4):417-23.
10.   Sharma D, Sharma P, Shastri S. Golden 60 minutes of newborn's life: Part 2: Term neonate. J Matern Fetal Neonatal Med. 2017;30(22):2728-33.
11.   Moon RY, Task Force On Sudden Infant Death S. SIDS and Other Sleep-Related Infant Deaths: Evidence Base for 2016 Updated Recommendations for a Safe Infant Sleeping Environment. Pediatrics. 2016;138(5).
12.   Jhun I, Mata DA, Nordio F, Lee M, Schwartz J, Zanobetti A. Ambient Temperature and Sudden Infant Death Syndrome in the United States. Epidemiology. 2017;28(5):728-34.
13.   Meier PP, Furman LM, Degenhardt M. Increased lactation risk for late preterm infants and mothers: evidence and management strategies to protect breastfeeding. J Midwifery Womens Health. 2007;52(6):579-87.
14.   Ponsonby AL, Dwyer T, Gibbons LE, Cochrane JA, Jones ME, McCall MJ. Thermal environment and sudden infant death syndrome: case-control study. BMJ. 1992;304(6822):277-82.
15.   Ponsonby AL, Dwyer T, Cochrane JA, Gibbons LE, Jones ME. Characteristics of the infant thermal environment in the control population of a case-control study of SIDS. J Paediatr Child Health. 1992;28 Suppl 1:S36-40.

16.	McLaren C, Null J, Quinn J. Heat stress from enclosed vehicles: moderate ambient temperatures cause significant temperature rise in enclosed vehicles. Pediatrics. 2005;116(1):e109-12.
17.	Goines L. The importance of quiet in the home: Teaching noise awareness to parents before the infant is discharged from the NICU. Neonatal Netw. 2008;27(3):171-6.
18.	Thomas KA, Spieker S. Sleep, Depression, and Fatigue in Late Postpartum. MCN Am J Matern Child Nurs. 2016;41(2):104-9.
19.	White-Traut RC, Rankin KM, Yoder J, Zawacki L, Campbell S, Kavanaugh K, et al. Relationship between mother-infant mutual dyadic responsiveness and premature infant development as measured by the Bayley III at 6weeks corrected age. Early Hum Dev. 2018;121:21-6.
20.	Tessier R, Charpak N, Giron M, Cristo M, de Calume ZF, Ruiz-Pelaez JG. Kangaroo Mother Care, home environment and father involvement in the first year of life: a randomized controlled study. Acta Paediatr. 2009;98(9):1444-50.
21.	Maitre NL, Key AP, Chorna OD, Slaughter JC, Matusz PJ, Wallace MT, et al. The Dual Nature of Early-Life Experience on Somatosensory Processing in the Human Infant Brain. Curr Biol. 2017;27(7):1048-54.
22.	Oras P, Thernstrom Blomqvist Y, Hedberg Nyqvist K, Gradin M, Rubertsson C, Hellstrom-Westas L, et al. Skin-to-skin contact is associated with earlier breastfeeding attainment in preterm infants. Acta Paediatr. 2016;105(7):783-9.
23.	Tuulari JJ, Scheinin NM, Lehtola S, Merisaari H, Saunavaara J, Parkkola R, et al. Neural correlates of gentle skin stroking in early infancy. Dev Cogn Neurosci. 2019;35:36-41.
24.	Sanchez-Solis M, Perez-Fernandez V, Bosch-Gimenez V, Quesada JJ, Garcia-Marcos L. Lung function gain in preterm infants with and without bronchopulmonary dysplasia. Pediatr Pulmonol. 2016;51(9):936-42.
25.	Langston C, Kida K, Reed M, Thurlbeck WM. Human lung growth in late gestation and in the neonate. Am Rev Respir Dis. 1984;129(4):607-13.
26.	Dobbing J, Sands J. Quantitative growth and development of human brain. Arch Dis Child. 1973;48(10):757-67.
27.	Aiello AE, Coulborn RM, Perez V, Larson EL. Effect of hand hygiene on infectious disease risk in the community setting: a meta-analysis. Am J Public Health. 2008;98(8):1372-81.
28.	Nicholson EG, Avadhanula V, Ferlic-Stark L, Patel K, Gincoo KE, Piedra PA. The Risk of Serious Bacterial Infection in Febrile Infants 0-90 Days of Life With a Respiratory Viral Infection. Pediatr Infect Dis J. 2019;38(4):355-61.
29.	Sauer CW, Boutin MA, Kim JH. Wide Variability in Caloric Density of Expressed Human Milk Can Lead to Major Underestimation or Overestimation of Nutrient Content. J Hum Lact. 2017;33(2):341-50.
30.	Kaiser JR, Bai S, Gibson N, Holland G, Lin TM, Swearingen CJ, et al. Association Between Transient Newborn Hypoglycemia and Fourth-Grade Achievement Test Proficiency: A Population-Based Study. JAMA Pediatr. 2015;169(10):913-21.

31.   Leung C, Chang WC, Yeh SJ. Hypernatremic dehydration due to concentrated infant formula: report of two cases. Pediatr Neonatol. 2009;50(2):70-3.
32.   Feldman-Winter L, Goldsmith JP, Committee On F, Newborn, Task Force On Sudden Infant Death S. Safe Sleep and Skin-to-Skin Care in the Neonatal Period for Healthy Term Newborns. Pediatrics. 2016;138(3).
33.   McInerny TK. Breastfeeding, early brain development, and epigenetics--getting children off to their best start. Breastfeed Med. 2014;9(7):333-4.
34.   Ballard O, Morrow AL. Human milk composition: nutrients and bioactive factors. Pediatr Clin North Am. 2013;60(1):49-74.
35.   Hassiotou F, Geddes DT. Immune cell-mediated protection of the mammary gland and the infant during breastfeeding. Adv Nutr. 2015;6(3):267-75.
36.   Wagner CL, Taylor SN, Johnson DD, Hollis BW. The role of vitamin D in pregnancy and lactation: emerging concepts. Womens Health (Lond). 2012;8(3):323-40.
37.   Wagner CL, Hollis BW, Kotsa K, Fakhoury H, Karras SN. Vitamin D administration during pregnancy as prevention for pregnancy, neonatal and postnatal complications. Rev Endocr Metab Disord. 2017;18(3):307-22.
38.   Pittard WB, 3rd, Geddes KM, Hulsey TC, Hollis BW. How much vitamin D for neonates? Am J Dis Child. 1991;145(10):1147-9.
39.   Taylor SN. ABM Clinical Protocol #29: Iron, Zinc, and Vitamin D Supplementation During Breastfeeding. Breastfeed Med. 2018;13(6):398-404.
40.   Milligan RA. Protein-protein interactions in the rigor actomyosin complex. Proc Natl Acad Sci U S A. 1996;93(1):21-6.
41.   Callahan S, Sejourne N, Denis A. Fatigue and breastfeeding: an inevitable partnership? J Hum Lact. 2006;22(2):182-7.
42.   Wambach KA. Maternal fatigue in breastfeeding primiparae during the first nine weeks postpartum. J Hum Lact. 1998;14(3):219-29.
43.   Lawrence RM, Lawrence RA. Breastfeeding: more than just good nutrition. Pediatr Rev. 2011;32(7):267-80.
44.   Dobbing J. Proceedings: Growth retardation and the human fetal brain. Arch Dis Child. 1973;48(10):828.
45.   Stiles J, Jernigan TL. The basics of brain development. Neuropsychol Rev. 2010;20(4):327-48.
46.   Tokariev A, Videman M, Palva JM, Vanhatalo S. Functional Brain Connectivity Develops Rapidly Around Term Age and Changes Between Vigilance States in the Human Newborn. Cereb Cortex. 2016;26(12):4540-50.
47.   Lopez J, Roffwarg HP, Dreher A, Bissette G, Karolewicz B, Shaffery JP. Rapid eye movement sleep deprivation decreases long-term potentiation stability and affects some glutamatergic signaling proteins during hippocampal development. Neuroscience. 2008;153(1):44-53.
48.   Maitre NL, Key AP. Quantitative assessment of cortical auditory-tactile processing in children with disabilities. J Vis Exp. 2014(83):e51054.
49.   Cascio CJ, Moore D, McGlone F. Social touch and human development. Dev Cogn Neurosci. 2019;35:5-11.

50.   Scher MS, Ludington-Hoe S, Kaffashi F, Johnson MW, Holditch-Davis D, Loparo KA. Neurophysiologic assessment of brain maturation after an 8-week trial of skin-to-skin contact on preterm infants. Clin Neurophysiol. 2009;120(10):1812-8.

51.   Schild SD, Mendelsohn MA, Plum A, Goldstein NA. Outcomes and Management of Infants Who Refer Newborn Hearing Screening. Ann Otol Rhinol Laryngol. 2023;132(12):1662-8.

52.   Amiel-Tison C, Ellison P. Birth asphyxia in the fullterm newborn: early assessment and outcome. Dev Med Child Neurol. 1986;28(5):671-82.

53.   Quinn F, Kearney PJ. French angles: a simple aid to neurodevelopmental examination. Ir Med J. 1989;82(3):131-2.

54.   Rossen LM. Quarterly provisional estimates for infant mortality, 2015-Quarter 2, 2017. National Center for Health Statistics, 20172017.

55.   You D, Hug L, Ejdemyr S, Idele P, Hogan D, Mathers C, et al. Global, regional, and national levels and trends in under-5 mortality between 1990 and 2015, with scenario-based projections to 2030: a systematic analysis by the UN Inter-agency Group for Child Mortality Estimation. Lancet. 2015;386(10010):2275-86.

56.   Auger N, Gilbert NL, Kaufman JS. Infant mortality at term in Canada: Impact of week of gestation. Early Hum Dev. 2016;100:43-7.

57.   Swanson JR, Sinkin RA. Transition from fetus to newborn. Pediatr Clin North Am. 2015;62(2):329-43.

58.   Law A, McCoy M, Lynen R, Curkendall SM, Gatwood J, Juneau PL, et al. The prevalence of complications and healthcare costs during pregnancy. J Med Econ. 2015;18(7):533-41.

59.   Jeyabalan A. Epidemiology of preeclampsia: impact of obesity. Nutr Rev. 2013;71 Suppl 1:S18-25.

60.   McDermott M, Miller EC, Rundek T, Hurn PD, Bushnell CD. Preeclampsia: Association With Posterior Reversible Encephalopathy Syndrome and Stroke. Stroke. 2018;49(3):524-30.

61.   Read JS, Klebanoff MA. Sexual intercourse during pregnancy and preterm delivery: effects of vaginal microorganisms. The Vaginal Infections and Prematurity Study Group. Am J Obstet Gynecol. 1993;168(2):514-9.

62.   Sayle AE, Savitz DA, Thorp JM, Jr., Hertz-Picciotto I, Wilcox AJ. Sexual activity during late pregnancy and risk of preterm delivery. Obstet Gynecol. 2001;97(2):283-9.

63.   Cleary GM, Wiswell TE. Meconium-stained amniotic fluid and the meconium aspiration syndrome. An update. Pediatr Clin North Am. 1998;45(3):511-29.

64.   Wyckoff MH, Aziz K, Escobedo MB, Kapadia VS, Kattwinkel J, Perlman JM, et al. Part 13: Neonatal Resuscitation: 2015 American Heart Association Guidelines Update for Cardiopulmonary Resuscitation and Emergency Cardiovascular Care. Circulation. 2015;132(18 Suppl 2):S543-60.

65.   Kattwinkel J, Perlman JM, Aziz K, Colby C, Fairchild K, Gallagher J, et al. Neonatal resuscitation: 2010 American Heart Association Guidelines for Cardiopulmonary Resuscitation and Emergency Cardiovascular Care. Pediatrics. 2010;126(5):e1400-13.

66.   American Heart A, American Academy of P. 2005 American Heart Association (AHA) guidelines for cardiopulmonary resuscitation (CPR) and emergency cardiovascular care (ECC) of pediatric and neonatal patients: neonatal resuscitation guidelines. Pediatrics. 2006;117(5):e1029-38.

67.   Perlman JM, Wyllie J, Kattwinkel J, Atkins DL, Chameides L, Goldsmith JP, et al. Part 11: Neonatal resuscitation: 2010 International Consensus on Cardiopulmonary Resuscitation and Emergency Cardiovascular Care Science With Treatment Recommendations. Circulation. 2010;122(16 Suppl 2):S516-38.

68.   de Jonge A, Geerts CC, van der Goes BY, Mol BW, Buitendijk SE, Nijhuis JG. Perinatal mortality and morbidity up to 28 days after birth among 743 070 low-risk planned home and hospital births: a cohort study based on three merged national perinatal databases. BJOG. 2015;122(5):720-8.

69.   Snowden JM, Tilden EL, Snyder J, Quigley B, Caughey AB, Cheng YW. Planned Out-of-Hospital Birth and Birth Outcomes. N Engl J Med. 2015;373(27):2642-53.

70.   Katheria AC, Lakshminrusimha S, Rabe H, McAdams R, Mercer JS. Placental transfusion: a review. J Perinatol. 2017;37(2):105-11.

71.   Rabe H, Reynolds G, Diaz-Rossello J. Early versus delayed umbilical cord clamping in preterm infants. Cochrane Database Syst Rev. 2004(4):CD003248.

72.   Sharma D. Golden 60 minutes of newborn's life: Part 1: Preterm neonate. J Matern Fetal Neonatal Med. 2017;30(22):2716-27.

73.   McDonald SJ, Middleton P, Dowswell T, Morris PS. Effect of timing of umbilical cord clamping of term infants on maternal and neonatal outcomes. Cochrane Database Syst Rev. 2013(7):CD004074.

74.   Safari K, Saeed AA, Hasan SS, Moghaddam-Banaem L. The effect of mother and newborn early skin-to-skin contact on initiation of breastfeeding, newborn temperature and duration of third stage of labor. Int Breastfeed J. 2018;13:32.

75.   Casper C, Sarapuk I, Pavlyshyn H. Regular and prolonged skin-to-skin contact improves short-term outcomes for very preterm infants: A dose-dependent intervention. Arch Pediatr. 2018;25(8):469-75.

76.   Feldman R, Rosenthal Z, Eidelman AI. Maternal-preterm skin-to-skin contact enhances child physiologic organization and cognitive control across the first 10 years of life. Biol Psychiatry. 2014;75(1):56-64.

77.   Harrison TM, Chen CY, Stein P, Brown R, Heathcock JC. Neonatal Skin-to-Skin Contact: Implications for Learning and Autonomic Nervous System Function in Infants With Congenital Heart Disease. Biol Res Nurs. 2019;21(3):296-306.

78.   Karimi FZ, Sadeghi R, Maleki-Saghooni N, Khadivzadeh T. The effect of mother-infant skin to skin contact on success and duration of first breastfeeding: A systematic review and meta-analysis. Taiwan J Obstet Gynecol. 2019;58(1):1-9.

79.   Matejcek A, Goldman RD. Treatment and prevention of ophthalmia neonatorum. Can Fam Physician. 2013;59(11):1187-90.

80.   Woods CR. Gonococcal infections in neonates and young children. Semin Pediatr Infect Dis. 2005;16(4):258-70.

81.   Araki S, Shirahata A. Vitamin K Deficiency Bleeding in Infancy. Nutrients. 2020;12(3).

82.   Shearer MJ. Vitamin K deficiency bleeding (VKDB) in early infancy. Blood Rev. 2009;23(2):49-59.

83.   Faridi MM, Rattan A, Ahmad SH. Omphalitis neonatorum. J Indian Med Assoc. 1993;91(11):283-5.

84.   Steer-Massaro C. Neonatal Omphalitis After Lotus Birth. J Midwifery Womens Health. 2020;65(2):271-5.

85.   Stewart D, Benitz W, Committee On F, Newborn. Umbilical Cord Care in the Newborn Infant. Pediatrics. 2016;138(3).

86.   Al-Shehri H. The Use of Alcohol versus Dry Care for the Umbilical Cord in Newborns: A Systematic Review and Meta-analysis of Randomized and Non-randomized Studies. Cureus. 2019;11(7):e5103.

87.   Jain L, Eaton DC. Physiology of fetal lung fluid clearance and the effect of labor. Semin Perinatol. 2006;30(1):34-43.

88.   Organization BotWH. Timing and Cummulative Probability of Neonatal Deaths. In: Genebra, editor.: World Health Organization; 2006.

89.   Phibbs CS, Baker LC, Caughey AB, Danielsen B, Schmitt SK, Phibbs RH. Level and volume of neonatal intensive care and mortality in very-low-birth-weight infants. N Engl J Med. 2007;356(21):2165-75.

90.   Benitz WE, Committee on F, Newborn AAoP. Hospital stay for healthy term newborn infants. Pediatrics. 2015;135(5):948-53.

91.   Thulier D. Challenging Expected Patterns of Weight Loss in Full-Term Breastfeeding Neonates Born by Cesarean. J Obstet Gynecol Neonatal Nurs. 2017;46(1):18-28.

92.   Mezzacappa MA, Ferreira BG. Excessive weight loss in exclusively breastfed full-term newborns in a Baby-Friendly Hospital. Rev Paul Pediatr. 2016;34(3):281-6.

93.   Mai CT, Riehle-Colarusso T, O'Halloran A, Cragan JD, Olney RS, Lin A, et al. Selected birth defects data from population-based birth defects surveillance programs in the United States, 2005-2009: Featuring critical congenital heart defects targeted for pulse oximetry screening. Birth Defects Res A Clin Mol Teratol. 2012;94(12):970-83.

94.   Eckersley L, Sadler L, Parry E, Finucane K, Gentles TL. Timing of diagnosis affects mortality in critical congenital heart disease. Arch Dis Child. 2016;101(6):516-20.

95.   Kemper AR, Mahle WT, Martin GR, Cooley WC, Kumar P, Morrow WR, et al. Strategies for implementing screening for critical congenital heart disease. Pediatrics. 2011;128(5):e1259-67.

96.   Wertheim-Tysarowska K, Gos M, Sykut-Cegielska J, Bal J. Genetic analysis in inherited metabolic disorders--from diagnosis to treatment. Own experience, current state of knowledge and perspectives. Dev Period Med. 2015;19(4):413-31.

97.   Mak CM, Lee HC, Chan AY, Lam CW. Inborn errors of metabolism and expanded newborn screening: review and update. Crit Rev Clin Lab Sci. 2013;50(6):142-62.

98.   Morton CC, Nance WE. Newborn hearing screening--a silent revolution. N Engl J Med. 2006;354(20):2151-64.

99.   Vohr B, Jodoin-Krauzyk J, Tucker R, Johnson MJ, Topol D, Ahlgren M. Early language outcomes of early-identified infants with permanent hearing loss at 12 to 16 months of age. Pediatrics. 2008;122(3):535-44.

100.   Vohr B, Jodoin-Krauzyk J, Tucker R, Topol D, Johnson MJ, Ahlgren M, et al. Expressive vocabulary of children with hearing loss in the first 2 years of life: impact of early intervention. J Perinatol. 2011;31(4):274-80.

101.   Vohr BR, Jodoin-Krauzyk J, Tucker R, Johnson MJ, Topol D, Ahlgren M. Results of newborn screening for hearing loss: effects on the family in the first 2 years of life. Arch Pediatr Adolesc Med. 2008;162(3):205-11.

102.   Vohr B, Topol D, Girard N, St Pierre L, Watson V, Tucker R. Language outcomes and service provision of preschool children with congenital hearing loss. Early Hum Dev. 2012;88(7):493-8.

103.   Jain L, Eaton DC. Alveolar fluid transport: a changing paradigm. Am J Physiol Lung Cell Mol Physiol. 2006;290(4):L646-L8.

104.   Jain L, Dudell GG. Respiratory transition in infants delivered by cesarean section. Semin Perinatol. 2006;30(5):296-304.

105.   Jha K, Nassar GN, Makker K. Transient Tachypnea of the Newborn. StatPearls. Treasure Island (FL)2020.

106.   Ladhani SN, Henderson KL, Muller-Pebody B, Ramsay ME, Riordan A. Risk of invasive bacterial infections by week of age in infants: prospective national surveillance, England, 2010-2017. Arch Dis Child. 2019;104(9):874-8.

107.   Stoll BJ, Hansen NI, Sanchez PJ, Faix RG, Poindexter BB, Van Meurs KP, et al. Early onset neonatal sepsis: the burden of group B Streptococcal and E. coli disease continues. Pediatrics. 2011;127(5):817-26.

108.   Vergnano S, Menson E, Kennea N, Embleton N, Russell AB, Watts T, et al. Neonatal infections in England: the NeonIN surveillance network. Arch Dis Child Fetal Neonatal Ed. 2011;96(1):F9-F14.

109.   Prevention of Group B Streptococcal Early-Onset Disease in Newborns: ACOG Committee Opinion, Number 782. Obstet Gynecol. 2019;134(1):e19-e40.

110.   Lubchenco LO, Bard H. Incidence of hypoglycemia in newborn infants classified by birth weight and gestational age. Pediatrics. 1971;47(5):831-8.

111.   Bromiker R, Perry A, Kasirer Y, Einav S, Klinger G, Levy-Khademi F. Early neonatal hypoglycemia: incidence of and risk factors. A cohort study using universal point of care screening. J Matern Fetal Neonatal Med. 2019;32(5):786-92.

112.   Harris DL, Weston PJ, Harding JE. Incidence of neonatal hypoglycemia in babies identified as at risk. J Pediatr. 2012;161(5):787-91.

113.   Ergaz Z, Ornoy A. Perinatal and early postnatal factors underlying developmental delay and disabilities. Dev Disabil Res Rev. 2011;17(2):59-70.

114.   Inder T. How low can I go? The impact of hypoglycemia on the immature brain. Pediatrics. 2008;122(2):440-1.

115.   Salhab WA, Wyckoff MH, Laptook AR, Perlman JM. Initial hypoglycemia and neonatal brain injury in term infants with severe fetal acidemia. Pediatrics. 2004;114(2):361-6.

116.   Palylyk-Colwell E, Campbell K. Oral Glucose Gel for Neonatal Hypoglycemia: A Review of Clinical Effectiveness, Cost-Effectiveness and Guidelines. CADTH Rapid Response Reports. Ottawa (ON)2018.

117.   Bhutani VK, Johnson L. Kernicterus in the 21st century: frequently asked questions. J Perinatol. 2009;29 Suppl 1:S20-4.
118.   Amiel-Tison C, Sureau C, Shnider SM. Cerebral handicap in full-term neonates related to the mechanical forces of labour. Baillieres Clin Obstet Gynaecol. 1988;2(1):145-65.
119.   Ahn ES, Jung MS, Lee YK, Ko SY, Shin SM, Hahn MH. Neonatal clavicular fracture: recent 10 year study. Pediatr Int. 2015;57(1):60-3.
120.   Basit H, Ali CDM, Madhani NB. Erb Palsy. StatPearls. Treasure Island (FL)2020.
121.   Chater M, Camfield P, Camfield C. Erb's palsy - Who is to blame and what will happen? Paediatr Child Health. 2004;9(8):556-60.
122.   Cha CI, Hong CK, Park MS, Yeo SG. Comparison of facial nerve paralysis in adults and children. Yonsei Med J. 2008;49(5):725-34.
123.   Laing JH, Harrison DH, Jones BM, Laing GJ. Is permanent congenital facial palsy caused by birth trauma? Arch Dis Child. 1996;74(1):56-8.
124.   Al Tawil K, Saleem N, Kadri H, Rifae MT, Tawakol H. Traumatic facial nerve palsy in newborns: is it always iatrogenic? Am J Perinatol. 2010;27(9):711-3.
125.   Walker NR, Mistry RK, Mazzoni T. Facial Nerve Palsy. StatPearls. Treasure Island (FL)2020.
126.   Techasatian L, Sanaphay V, Paopongsawan P, Schachner LA. Neonatal Birthmarks: A Prospective Survey in 1000 Neonates. Glob Pediatr Health. 2019;6:2333794X19835668.
127.   Reginatto FP, Villa DD, Cestari TF. Benign skin disease with pustules in the newborn. An Bras Dermatol. 2016;91(2):124-34.
128.   Czinn SJ, Blanchard S. Gastroesophageal reflux disease in neonates and infants : when and how to treat. Paediatr Drugs. 2013;15(1):19-27.
129.   Rybak A, Pesce M, Thapar N, Borrelli O. Gastro-Esophageal Reflux in Children. Int J Mol Sci. 2017;18(8).
130.   Vaezi MF, Yang YX, Howden CW. Complications of Proton Pump Inhibitor Therapy. Gastroenterology. 2017;153(1):35-48.
131.   Host A. Cow's milk protein allergy and intolerance in infancy. Some clinical, epidemiological and immunological aspects. Pediatr Allergy Immunol. 1994;5(5 Suppl):1-36.
132.   Schrander JJ, van den Bogart JP, Forget PP, Schrander-Stumpel CT, Kuijten RH, Kester AD. Cow's milk protein intolerance in infants under 1 year of age: a prospective epidemiological study. Eur J Pediatr. 1993;152(8):640-4.
133.   Host A, Halken S. Cow's milk allergy: where have we come from and where are we going? Endocr Metab Immune Disord Drug Targets. 2014;14(1):2-8.
134.   Sambrook J. Incidence of cow's milk protein allergy. Br J Gen Pract. 2016;66(651):512.
135.   Schrander JJ, Dellevoet JJ, Arends JW, Forget PP, Kuijten R. Small intestinal mucosa IgE plasma cells and specific anti-cow milk IgE in children with cow milk protein intolerance. Ann Allergy. 1993;70(5):406-9.
136.   Zeiger RS, Sampson HA, Bock SA, Burks AW, Jr., Harden K, Noone S, et al. Soy allergy in infants and children with IgE-associated cow's milk allergy. J Pediatr. 1999;134(5):614-22.

137.   Ahn KM, Han YS, Nam SY, Park HY, Shin MY, Lee SI. Prevalence of soy protein hypersensitivity in cow's milk protein-sensitive children in Korea. J Korean Med Sci. 2003;18(4):473-7.

138.   Johnson JD, Cocker K, Chang E. Infantile Colic: Recognition and Treatment. Am Fam Physician. 2015;92(7):577-82.

139.   Roberts DM, Ostapchuk M, O'Brien JG. Infantile colic. Am Fam Physician. 2004;70(4):735-40.

140.   Lee C, Barr RG, Catherine N, Wicks A. Age-related incidence of publicly reported shaken baby syndrome cases: is crying a trigger for shaking? J Dev Behav Pediatr. 2007;28(4):288-93.

141.   Kim H, Sitarik AR, Woodcroft K, Johnson CC, Zoratti E. Birth Mode, Breastfeeding, Pet Exposure, and Antibiotic Use: Associations With the Gut Microbiome and Sensitization in Children. Curr Allergy Asthma Rep. 2019;19(4):22.

142.   Arvola T, Ruuska T, Keranen J, Hyoty H, Salminen S, Isolauri E. Rectal bleeding in infancy: clinical, allergological, and microbiological examination. Pediatrics. 2006;117(4):e760-8.

143.   Fiess A, Kolb-Keerl R, Schuster AK, Knuf M, Kirchhof B, Muether PS, et al. Prevalence and associated factors of strabismus in former preterm and full-term infants between 4 and 10 Years of age. BMC Ophthalmol. 2017;17(1):228.

144.   Yang Y, Wang C, Gan Y, Jiang H, Fu W, Cao S, et al. Maternal smoking during pregnancy and the risk of strabismus in offspring: a meta-analysis. Acta Ophthalmol. 2019;97(4):353-63.

145.   Michaelides M, Moore AT. The genetics of strabismus. J Med Genet. 2004;41(9):641-6.

146.   Glass HC, Costarino AT, Stayer SA, Brett CM, Cladis F, Davis PJ. Outcomes for extremely premature infants. Anesth Analg. 2015;120(6):1337-51.

147.   Dammann O, Naples M, Bednarek F, Shah B, Kuban KC, O'Shea TM, et al. SNAP-II and SNAPPE-II and the risk of structural and functional brain disorders in extremely low gestational age newborns: the ELGAN study. Neonatology. 2010;97(2):71-82.

148.   Zysman-Colman Z, Tremblay GM, Bandeali S, Landry JS. Bronchopulmonary dysplasia - trends over three decades. Paediatr Child Health. 2013;18(2):86-90.

149.   Dammann O, Leviton A. Brain damage in preterm newborns: might enhancement of developmentally regulated endogenous protection open a door for prevention? Pediatrics. 1999;104(3 Pt 1):541-50.

150.   Woythaler M. Neurodevelopmental outcomes of the late preterm infant. Semin Fetal Neonatal Med. 2019;24(1):54-9.

151.   Mally PV, Bailey S, Hendricks-Munoz KD. Clinical issues in the management of late preterm infants. Curr Probl Pediatr Adolesc Health Care. 2010;40(9):218-33.

152.   Wyckoff MH. Initial resuscitation and stabilization of the periviable neonate: the Golden-Hour approach. Semin Perinatol. 2014;38(1):12-6.

153.   Vohr BR, Wright LL, Dusick AM, Perritt R, Poole WK, Tyson JE, et al. Center differences and outcomes of extremely low birth weight infants. Pediatrics. 2004;113(4):781-9.

154.   Alleman BW, Bell EF, Li L, Dagle JM, Smith PB, Ambalavanan N, et al. Individual and center-level factors affecting mortality among extremely low birth weight infants. Pediatrics. 2013;132(1):e175-84.

155.   Moore GP, Lemyre B, Barrowman N, Daboval T. Neurodevelopmental outcomes at 4 to 8 years of children born at 22 to 25 weeks' gestational age: a meta-analysis. JAMA Pediatr. 2013;167(10):967-74.

156.   McCormick AE. Infant Mortality and Child-Naming: A Genealogical Exploration of American Trends. The Journal of Public and Professional Sociology. 2010;3(1).

157.   Brosco JP. The early history of the infant mortality rate in America: "A reflection upon the past and a prophecy of the future". Pediatrics. 1999;103(2):478-85.

158.   Lawn JE, Cousens S, Zupan J, Lancet Neonatal Survival Steering T. 4 million neonatal deaths: when? Where? Why? Lancet. 2005;365(9462):891-900.

159.   Lee KS. Infant mortality decline in the late 19th and early 20th centuries: the role of market milk. Perspect Biol Med. 2007;50(4):585-602.

160.   Matsuura H. State constitutional commitment to health and health care and population health outcomes: evidence from historical US data. Am J Public Health. 2015;105 Suppl 3:e48-54.

161.   Wright JR, Jr. A Fresh Look at the History of SIDS. Acad Forensic Pathol. 2017;7(2):146-62.

162.   Division of Reproductive Health NCfCDPaHP. Sudden Unexpected Infant Death and Sudden Infant Death Syndrome. U.S. Department of Health & Human Services; 2020.

163.   Lavezzi AM, Ottaviani G, Matturri L. Developmental alterations of the auditory brainstem centers--pathogenetic implications in Sudden Infant Death Syndrome. J Neurol Sci. 2015;357(1-2):257-63.

164.   Erck Lambert AB, Parks SE, Shapiro-Mendoza CK. National and State Trends in Sudden Unexpected Infant Death: 1990-2015. Pediatrics. 2018;141(3).

165.   Carlberg MM, Shapiro-Mendoza CK, Goodman M. Maternal and infant characteristics associated with accidental suffocation and strangulation in bed in US infants. Matern Child Health J. 2012;16(8):1594-601.

166.   Hunt CE. Ontogeny of autonomic regulation in late preterm infants born at 34-37 weeks postmenstrual age. Semin Perinatol. 2006;30(2):73-6.

167.   Malloy MH, Hoffman HJ. Prematurity, sudden infant death syndrome, and age of death. Pediatrics. 1995;96(3 Pt 1):464-71.

168.   Filiano JJ, Kinney HC. A perspective on neuropathologic findings in victims of the sudden infant death syndrome: the triple-risk model. Biol Neonate. 1994;65(3-4):194-7.

169.   Tieder JS, Bonkowsky JL, Etzel RA, Franklin WH, Gremse DA, Herman B, et al. Brief Resolved Unexplained Events (Formerly Apparent Life-Threatening Events) and Evaluation of Lower-Risk Infants: Executive Summary. Pediatrics. 2016;137(5).

170.   Kiechl-Kohlendorfer U, Hof D, Peglow UP, Traweger-Ravanelli B, Kiechl S. Epidemiology of apparent life threatening events. Arch Dis Child. 2005;90(3):297-300.

171.   Fleming PJ, Azaz Y, Wigfield R. Development of thermoregulation in infancy: possible implications for SIDS. J Clin Pathol. 1992;45(11 Suppl):17-9.
172.   Hauck FR, Herman SM, Donovan M, Iyasu S, Merrick Moore C, Donoghue E, et al. Sleep environment and the risk of sudden infant death syndrome in an urban population: the Chicago Infant Mortality Study. Pediatrics. 2003;111(5 Pt 2):1207-14.
173.   Sawczenko A, Fleming PJ. Thermal stress, sleeping position, and the sudden infant death syndrome. Sleep. 1996;19(10 Suppl):S267-70.
174.   Committee on F, Newborn. American Academy of P. Apnea, sudden infant death syndrome, and home monitoring. Pediatrics. 2003;111(4 Pt 1):914-7.
175.   Logan JW, et al Journal of Pediatrics, 2024.
176.   Schieve LA, Boulet SL, Kogan MD, Van Naarden-Braun K, Boyle CA. A population-based assessment of the health, functional status, and consequent family impact among children with Down syndrome. Disabil Health J. 2011;4(2):68-77.
177.   Van Naarden Braun K, Christensen D, Doernberg N, Schieve L, Rice C, Wiggins L, et al. Trends in the prevalence of autism spectrum disorder, cerebral palsy, hearing loss, intellectual disability, and vision impairment, metropolitan atlanta, 1991-2010. PLoS One. 2015;10(4):e0124120.
178.   Schieve LA, Clayton HB, Durkin MS, Wingate MS, Drews-Botsch C. Comparison of Perinatal Risk Factors Associated with Autism Spectrum Disorder (ASD), Intellectual Disability (ID), and Co-occurring ASD and ID. J Autism Dev Disord. 2015;45(8):2361-72.
179.   Aarnoudse-Moens CS, Weisglas-Kuperus N, van Goudoever JB, Oosterlaan J. Meta-analysis of neurobehavioral outcomes in very preterm and/or very low birth weight children. Pediatrics. 2009;124(2):717-28.
180.   Aarnoudse-Moens CS, Smidts DP, Oosterlaan J, Duivenvoorden HJ, Weisglas-Kuperus N. Executive function in very preterm children at early school age. J Abnorm Child Psychol. 2009;37(7):981-93.
181.   Johnson S, Evans TA, Draper ES, Field DJ, Manktelow BN, Marlow N, et al. Neurodevelopmental outcomes following late and moderate prematurity: a population-based cohort study. Arch Dis Child Fetal Neonatal Ed. 2015;100(4):F301-8.
182.   Thornberg E, Thiringer K, Odeback A, Milsom I. Birth asphyxia: incidence, clinical course and outcome in a Swedish population. Acta Paediatr. 1995;84(8):927-32.
183.   Nolan R, Luther B, Young P, Murphy NA. Differing perceptions regarding quality of life and inpatient treatment goals for children with severe disabilities. Acad Pediatr. 2014;14(6):574-80.
184.   Jardine J, Glinianaia SV, McConachie H, Embleton ND, Rankin J. Self-reported quality of life of young children with conditions from early infancy: a systematic review. Pediatrics. 2014;134(4):e1129-48.
185.   Dickinson HO, Parkinson KN, Ravens-Sieberer U, Schirripa G, Thyen U, Arnaud C, et al. Self-reported quality of life of 8-12-year-old children with cerebral palsy: a cross-sectional European study. Lancet. 2007;369(9580):2171-8.

186.   Young NL, Rochon TG, McCormick A, Law M, Wedge JH, Fehlings D. The health and quality of life outcomes among youth and young adults with cerebral palsy. Arch Phys Med Rehabil. 2010;91(1):143-8.

187.   Presson AP, Partyka G, Jensen KM, Devine OJ, Rasmussen SA, McCabe LL, et al. Current estimate of Down Syndrome population prevalence in the United States. J Pediatr. 2013;163(4):1163-8.

188.   Graves RJ, Graff JC, Esbensen AJ, Hathaway DK, Wan JY, Wicks MN. Measuring Health-Related Quality of Life of Adults With Down Syndrome. Am J Intellect Dev Disabil. 2016;121(4):312-26.

189.   Natoli JL, Ackerman DL, McDermott S, Edwards JG. Prenatal diagnosis of Down syndrome: a systematic review of termination rates (1995-2011). Prenat Diagn. 2012;32(2):142-53.

190.   Grossman TB, Chasen ST. Abortion for Fetal Genetic Abnormalities: Type of Abnormality and Gestational Age at Diagnosis. AJP Rep. 2020;10(1):e87-e92.

191.   Evans MI, Littman L, Richter R, Richter K, Hume RF, Jr. Selective reduction for multifetal pregnancy. Early opinions revisited. J Reprod Med. 1997;42(12):771-7.

192.   Janvier A, Couture E, Deschenes M, Nadeau S, Barrington K, Lantos J. Health care professionals' attitudes about pregnancy termination for different fetal anomalies. Paediatr Child Health. 2012;17(8):e86-8.

193.   Glinianaia SV, Rankin J, Tan J, Loane M, Garne E, Cavero-Carbonell C, et al. Ten-year survival of children with trisomy 13 or trisomy 18: a multi-registry European cohort study. Arch Dis Child. 2023;108(6):461-7.

194.   Peterson JK, Kochilas LK, Catton KG, Moller JH, Setty SP. Long-Term Outcomes of Children With Trisomy 13 and 18 After Congenital Heart Disease Interventions. Ann Thorac Surg. 2017;103(6):1941-9.

195.   Bruns DA, Martinez A. An analysis of cardiac defects and surgical interventions in 84 cases with full trisomy 18. Am J Med Genet A. 2016;170A(2):337-43.

196.   Cooper DS, Riggs KW, Zafar F, Jacobs JP, Hill KD, Pasquali SK, et al. Cardiac Surgery in Patients With Trisomy 13 and 18: An Analysis of The Society of Thoracic Surgeons Congenital Heart Surgery Database. J Am Heart Assoc. 2019;8(13):e012349.

197.   Janvier A, Farlow B, Barrington K. Cardiac surgery for children with trisomies 13 and 18: Where are we now? Semin Perinatol. 2016;40(4):254-60.

198.   Smeeth L, Cook C, Fombonne PE, Heavey L, Rodrigues LC, Smith PG, et al. Rate of first recorded diagnosis of autism and other pervasive developmental disorders in United Kingdom general practice, 1988 to 2001. BMC Med. 2004;2:39.

199.   Phadke VK, Bednarczyk RA, Salmon DA, Omer SB. Association Between Vaccine Refusal and Vaccine-Preventable Diseases in the United States: A Review of Measles and Pertussis. JAMA. 2016;315(11):1149-58.

200.   Carrillo-Marquez M, White L. Current controversies in childhood vaccination. S D Med. 2013;Spec no:46-51.

201.   Munoz FM. Safer Pertussis Vaccines for Children: Trading Efficacy for Safety. Pediatrics. 2018;142(1).

202.   Chatterjee A, O'Keefe C. Current controversies in the USA regarding vaccine safety. Expert Rev Vaccines. 2010;9(5):497-502.

203.   Maglione MA, Das L, Raaen L, Smith A, Chari R, Newberry S, et al. Safety of vaccines used for routine immunization of U.S. children: a systematic review. Pediatrics. 2014;134(2):325-37.

204.   Doja A. Genetics and the myth of vaccine encephalopathy. Paediatr Child Health. 2008;13(7):597-9.

205.   Miller D, Madge N, Diamond J, Wadsworth J, Ross E. Pertussis immunisation and serious acute neurological illnesses in children. BMJ. 1993;307(6913):1171-6.

206.   Madge N, Diamond J, Miller D, Ross E, McManus C, Wadsworth J, et al. The National Childhood Encephalopathy study: a 10-year follow-up. A report on the medical, social, behavioural and educational outcomes after serious, acute, neurological illness in early childhood. Dev Med Child Neurol Suppl. 1993;68:1-118.

207.   Geier DA, Geier MR. Serious neurological conditions following pertussis immunization: an analysis of endotoxin levels, the vaccine adverse events reporting system (VAERS) database and literature review. Pediatr Rehabil. 2002;5(3):177-82.

208.   Madsen KM, Hviid A, Vestergaard M, Schendel D, Wohlfahrt J, Thorsen P, et al. A population-based study of measles, mumps, and rubella vaccination and autism. N Engl J Med. 2002;347(19):1477-82.

209.   Wilson K, Mills E, Ross C, McGowan J, Jadad A. Association of autistic spectrum disorder and the measles, mumps, and rubella vaccine: a systematic review of current epidemiological evidence. Arch Pediatr Adolesc Med. 2003;157(7):628-34.

210.   Smeeth L, Cook C, Fombonne E, Heavey L, Rodrigues LC, Smith PG, et al. MMR vaccination and pervasive developmental disorders: a case-control study. Lancet. 2004;364(9438):963-9.

211.   Honda H, Shimizu Y, Rutter M. No effect of MMR withdrawal on the incidence of autism: a total population study. J Child Psychol Psychiatry. 2005;46(6):572-9.

212.   Uchiyama T, Kurosawa M, Inaba Y. MMR-vaccine and regression in autism spectrum disorders: negative results presented from Japan. J Autism Dev Disord. 2007;37(2):210-7.

213.   Patja A, Davidkin I, Kurki T, Kallio MJ, Valle M, Peltola H. Serious adverse events after measles-mumps-rubella vaccination during a fourteen-year prospective follow-up. Pediatr Infect Dis J. 2000;19(12):1127-34.

214.   Taylor LE, Swerdfeger AL, Eslick GD. Vaccines are not associated with autism: an evidence-based meta-analysis of case-control and cohort studies. Vaccine. 2014;32(29):3623-9.

215.   Rice CE, Rosanoff M, Dawson G, Durkin MS, Croen LA, Singer A, et al. Evaluating Changes in the Prevalence of the Autism Spectrum Disorders (ASDs). Public Health Rev. 2012;34(2):1-22.

216.   Georgieff MK. Nutrition and the developing brain: nutrient priorities and measurement. Am J Clin Nutr. 2007;85(2):614S-20S.

217.   Allotey J, Zamora J, Cheong-See F, Kalidindi M, Arroyo-Manzano D, Asztalos E, et al. Cognitive, motor, behavioural and academic performances of

children born preterm: a meta-analysis and systematic review involving 64 061 children. BJOG. 2018;125(1):16-25.

218.   Ravishankar S, Redline RW. The placenta. Handb Clin Neurol. 2019;162:57-66.

219.   Li H, Saucedo-Cuevas L, Shresta S, Gleeson JG. The Neurobiology of Zika Virus. Neuron. 2016;92(5):949-58.

220.   Hagberg H, Mallard C. Effect of inflammation on central nervous system development and vulnerability. Curr Opin Neurol. 2005;18(2):117-23.

221.   Andreoli V, Sprovieri F. Genetic Aspects of Susceptibility to Mercury Toxicity: An Overview. Int J Environ Res Public Health. 2017;14(1).

222.   Tuteja N, Tuteja R. Unraveling DNA repair in human: molecular mechanisms and consequences of repair defect. Crit Rev Biochem Mol Biol. 2001;36(3):261-90.

223.   Davies E, Connolly DJ, Mordekar SR. Encephalopathy in children: an approach to assessment and management. Arch Dis Child. 2012;97(5):452-8.

224.   Milev MP, Grout ME, Saint-Dic D, Cheng YH, Glass IA, Hale CJ, et al. Mutations in TRAPPC12 Manifest in Progressive Childhood Encephalopathy and Golgi Dysfunction. Am J Hum Genet. 2017;101(2):291-9.

225.   Stromme P, Kanavin OJ, Abdelnoor M, Woldseth B, Rootwelt T, Diderichsen J, et al. Incidence rates of progressive childhood encephalopathy in Oslo, Norway: a population based study. BMC Pediatr. 2007;7:25.

226.   Tam J, Tran D, Bettinger JA, Moore D, Sauve L, Jadavji T, et al. Review of pediatric encephalitis and encephalopathy cases following immunization reported to the Canadian Immunization Monitoring Program Active (IMPACT) from 1992 to 2012. Vaccine. 2020;38(28):4457-63.

227.   Babenko O, Kovalchuk I, Metz GA. Stress-induced perinatal and transgenerational epigenetic programming of brain development and mental health. Neurosci Biobehav Rev. 2015;48:70-91.

228.   Weber-Stadlbauer U. Epigenetic and transgenerational mechanisms in infection-mediated neurodevelopmental disorders. Transl Psychiatry. 2017;7(5):e1113.

229.   Knudson AG, Jr. Mutation and cancer: statistical study of retinoblastoma. Proc Natl Acad Sci U S A. 1971;68(4):820-3.

230.   Folstein S, Rutter M. Infantile autism: a genetic study of 21 twin pairs. J Child Psychol Psychiatry. 1977;18(4):297-321.

231.   Folstein S, Rutter M. Genetic influences and infantile autism. Nature. 1977;265(5596):726-8.

232.   Brown NJ, Berkovic SF, Scheffer IE. Vaccination, seizures and 'vaccine damage'. Curr Opin Neurol. 2007;20(2):181-7.

233.   Kimmel SR. Vaccine adverse events: separating myth from reality. Am Fam Physician. 2002;66(11):2113-20.

234.   Roush SW, Murphy TV, Vaccine-Preventable Disease Table Working G. Historical comparisons of morbidity and mortality for vaccine-preventable diseases in the United States. JAMA. 2007;298(18):2155-63.

235.   Chang CJ, Tu YK, Chen PC, Yang HY. Occupational Exposure to Talc Increases the Risk of Lung Cancer: A Meta-Analysis of Occupational Cohort Studies. Can Respir J. 2017;2017:1270608.
236.   Whysner J, Mohan M. Perineal application of talc and cornstarch powders: evaluation of ovarian cancer risk. Am J Obstet Gynecol. 2000;182(3):720-4.
237.   Sarkadi A, Kristiansson R, Oberklaid F, Bremberg S. Fathers' involvement and children's developmental outcomes: a systematic review of longitudinal studies. Acta Paediatr. 2008;97(2):153-8.
238.   Alio AP, Salihu HM, Kornosky JL, Richman AM, Marty PJ. Feto-infant health and survival: does paternal involvement matter? Matern Child Health J. 2010;14(6):931-7.
239.   Alio AP, Mbah AK, Kornosky JL, Wathington D, Marty PJ, Salihu HM. Assessing the impact of paternal involvement on racial/ethnic disparities in infant mortality rates. J Community Health. 2011;36(1):63-8.
240.   Flouri E, Buchanan A. The role of father involvement in children's later mental health. J Adolesc. 2003;26(1):63-78.
241.   Sethna V, Perry E, Domoney J, Iles J, Psychogiou L, Rowbotham NEL, et al. Father-Child Interactions at 3 Months and 24 Months: Contributions to Children's Cognitive Development at 24 Months. Infant Ment Health J. 2017;38(3):378-90.
242.   Lee SJ, Sanchez DT, Grogan-Kaylor A, Lee JY, Albuja A. Father Early Engagement Behaviors and Infant Low Birth Weight. Matern Child Health J. 2018;22(10):1407-17.
243.   Gaudino JA, Jr., Jenkins B, Rochat RW. No fathers' names: a risk factor for infant mortality in the State of Georgia, USA. Soc Sci Med. 1999;48(2):253-65.
244.   Pearlstein T, Howard M, Salisbury A, Zlotnick C. Postpartum depression. Am J Obstet Gynecol. 2009;200(4):357-64.
245.   Silva CS, Lima MC, Sequeira-de-Andrade LAS, Oliveira JS, Monteiro JS, Lima NMS, et al. Association between postpartum depression and the practice of exclusive breastfeeding in the first three months of life. J Pediatr (Rio J). 2017;93(4):356-64.
246.   Robertson NJ, Kendall GS, Thayyil S. Techniques for therapeutic hypothermia during transport and in hospital for perinatal asphyxial encephalopathy. Semin Fetal Neonatal Med. 2010;15(5):276-86.
247.   Li MX, Sun G, Neubauer H. Change in the body temperature of healthy term infant over the first 72 hours of life. J Zhejiang Univ Sci. 2004;5(4):486-93.
248.   Puopolo KM, Draper D, Wi S, Newman TB, Zupancic J, Lieberman E, et al. Estimating the probability of neonatal early-onset infection on the basis of maternal risk factors. Pediatrics. 2011;128(5):e1155-63.
249.   Stoll BJ, Hansen N, Fanaroff AA, Wright LL, Carlo WA, Ehrenkranz RA, et al. Late-onset sepsis in very low birth weight neonates: the experience of the NICHD Neonatal Research Network. Pediatrics. 2002;110(2 Pt 1):285-91.
250.   Perez GF, Pancham K, Huseni S, Jain A, Rodriguez-Martinez CE, Preciado D, et al. Rhinovirus-induced airway cytokines and respiratory morbidity in severely premature children. Pediatr Allergy Immunol. 2015;26(2):145-52.
251.   Chuang YY, Huang YC. Enteroviral infection in neonates. J Microbiol Immunol Infect. 2019;52(6):851-7.

252.   Del Vecchio A, Ferrara T, Maglione M, Capasso L, Raimondi F. New perspectives in Respiratory Syncitial Virus infection. J Matern Fetal Neonatal Med. 2013;26 Suppl 2:55-9.

253.   Beigi RH, Wiesenfeld HC, Landers DV, Simhan HN. High rate of severe fetal outcomes associated with maternal parvovirus b19 infection in pregnancy. Infect Dis Obstet Gynecol. 2008;2008:524601.

254.   Okoli GN, Otete HE, Beck CR, Nguyen-Van-Tam JS. Use of neuraminidase inhibitors for rapid containment of influenza: a systematic review and meta-analysis of individual and household transmission studies. PLoS One. 2014;9(12):e113633.

255.   McGirr A, Fisman DN. Duration of pertussis immunity after DTaP immunization: a meta-analysis. Pediatrics. 2015;135(2):331-43.

256.   Mirbeyk M, Saghazadeh A, Rezaei N. A systematic review of pregnant women with COVID-19 and their neonates. Arch Gynecol Obstet. 2021;304(1):5-38.

257.   Bhuiyan MU, Stiboy E, Hassan MZ, Chan M, Islam MS, Haider N, et al. Epidemiology of COVID-19 infection in young children under five years: A systematic review and meta-analysis. Vaccine. 2021;39(4):667-77.

258.   Nehra D, Goldstein AM. Intestinal malrotation: varied clinical presentation from infancy through adulthood. Surgery. 2011;149(3):386-93.

259.   Leung AK, Sauve RS. Breastfeeding and breast milk jaundice. J R Soc Health. 1989;109(6):213-7.

260.   Cunningham MW. Pathogenesis of group A streptococcal infections. Clin Microbiol Rev. 2000;13(3):470-511.

261.   Glass HC. Hypoxic-Ischemic Encephalopathy and Other Neonatal Encephalopathies. Continuum (Minneap Minn). 2018;24(1, Child Neurology):57-71.

262.   Harris BS, Bishop KC, Kemeny HR, Walker JS, Rhee E, Kuller JA. Risk Factors for Birth Defects. Obstet Gynecol Surv. 2017;72(2):123-35.

263.   Rynn L, J Cragan, A Correa. Division of Birth Defects and Developmental Disabilities. In: Disabilities DoBDaD, editor. MMWR Weekly: National Center on Birth Defects and Developmental Disabilities, CDC.,; January 11, 2008. p. 1-5.

264.   Ludvigsson JF, Neovius M, Soderling J, Gudbjornsdottir S, Svensson AM, Franzen S, et al. Periconception glycaemic control in women with type 1 diabetes and risk of major birth defects: population based cohort study in Sweden. BMJ. 2018;362:k2638.

265.   Basu M, Zhu JY, LaHaye S, Majumdar U, Jiao K, Han Z, et al. Epigenetic mechanisms underlying maternal diabetes-associated risk of congenital heart disease. JCI Insight. 2017;2(20).

266.   St Louis AM, Kim K, Browne ML, Liu G, Liberman RF, Nembhard WN, et al. Prevalence trends of selected major birth defects: A multi-state population-based retrospective study, United States, 1999 to 2007. Birth Defects Res. 2017;109(18):1442-50.

267.   Parker SE, Mai CT, Canfield MA, Rickard R, Wang Y, Meyer RE, et al. Updated National Birth Prevalence estimates for selected birth defects in the United States, 2004-2006. Birth Defects Res A Clin Mol Teratol. 2010;88(12):1008-16.

268.   Marden PM, Smith DW, McDonald MJ. Congenital Anomalies in the Newborn Infant, Including Minor Variations. A Study of 4,412 Babies by Surface

Examination for Anomalies and Buccal Smear for Sex Chromatin. J Pediatr. 1964;64:357-71.

269.   Sawers N, Jewsbury H, Ali N. Diagnosis and management of childhood squints: investigation and examination with reference to red flags and referral letters. Br J Gen Pract. 2017;67(654):42-3.

270.   Khitri MR. Corneal Opacities in the Neonate. Neoreviews. 2018;19(No. 5):e269.

271.   Tanaka SA, Mahabir RC, Jupiter DC, Menezes JM. Updating the epidemiology of cleft lip with or without cleft palate. Plast Reconstr Surg. 2012;129(3):511e-8e.

272.   Wyszynski DF, Duffy DL, Beaty TH. Maternal cigarette smoking and oral clefts: a meta-analysis. Cleft Palate Craniofac J. 1997;34(3):206-10.

273.   Nunez-Castruita A, Lopez-Serna N. Low-set ears and associated anomalies in human foetuses. Int J Pediatr Otorhinolaryngol. 2018;104:126-33.

274.   Roth DA, Hildesheimer M, Bardenstein S, Goidel D, Reichman B, Maayan-Metzger A, et al. Preauricular skin tags and ear pits are associated with permanent hearing impairment in newborns. Pediatrics. 2008;122(4):e884-90.

275.   Smith CJF, Friedlander SF, Guma M, Kavanaugh A, Chambers CD. Infantile Hemangiomas: An Updated Review on Risk Factors, Pathogenesis, and Treatment. Birth Defects Res. 2017;109(11):809-15.

276.   Roche AF. Clinodactyly and brachymesophalangia of the fifth finger. Acta Paediatr. 1961;50:387-91.

277.   Delgadillo D, 3rd, Adams NS, Girotto JA. Supernumerary Digits of the Hand. Eplasty. 2016;16:ic3.

278.   Eaton CJ, Lister GD. Syndactyly. Hand Clin. 1990;6(4):555-75.

279.   Malik S. Syndactyly: phenotypes, genetics and current classification. Eur J Hum Genet. 2012;20(8):817-24.

280.   Bleck EE. Metatarsus adductus: classification and relationship to outcomes of treatment. J Pediatr Orthop. 1983;3(1):2-9.

281.   Farsetti P, Weinstein SL, Ponseti IV. The long-term functional and radiographic outcomes of untreated and non-operatively treated metatarsus adductus. J Bone Joint Surg Am. 1994;76(2):257-65.

282.   Anand A, Sala DA. Clubfoot: etiology and treatment. Indian J Orthop. 2008;42(1):22-8.

283.   Clinical practice guideline: early detection of developmental dysplasia of the hip. Committee on Quality Improvement, Subcommittee on Developmental Dysplasia of the Hip. American Academy of Pediatrics. Pediatrics. 2000;105(4 Pt 1):896-905.

284.   Garne E. Atrial and ventricular septal defects - epidemiology and spontaneous closure. J Matern Fetal Neonatal Med. 2006;19(5):271-6.

285.   Minette MS, Sahn DJ. Ventricular septal defects. Circulation. 2006;114(20):2190-7.

286.   Zee RS, Herbst KW, Kim C, McKenna PH, Bentley T, Cooper CS, et al. Urinary tract infections in children with prenatal hydronephrosis: A risk assessment from the Society for Fetal Urology Hydronephrosis Registry. J Pediatr Urol. 2016;12(4):261 e1-7.

287.   Chen MJ, Karaviti LP, Roth DR, Schlomer BJ. Birth prevalence of hypospadias and hypospadias risk factors in newborn males in the United States from 1997 to 2012. J Pediatr Urol. 2018;14(5):425 e1- e7.
288.   Bhimani AD, Selner AN, Patel JB, Hobbs JG, Esfahani DR, Behbahani M, et al. Pediatric tethered cord release: an epidemiological and postoperative complication analysis. J Spine Surg. 2019;5(3):337-50.

www.ingramcontent.com/pod-product-compliance
Lightning Source LLC
Chambersburg PA
CBHW030252130626
46549CB00002B/493